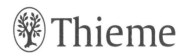

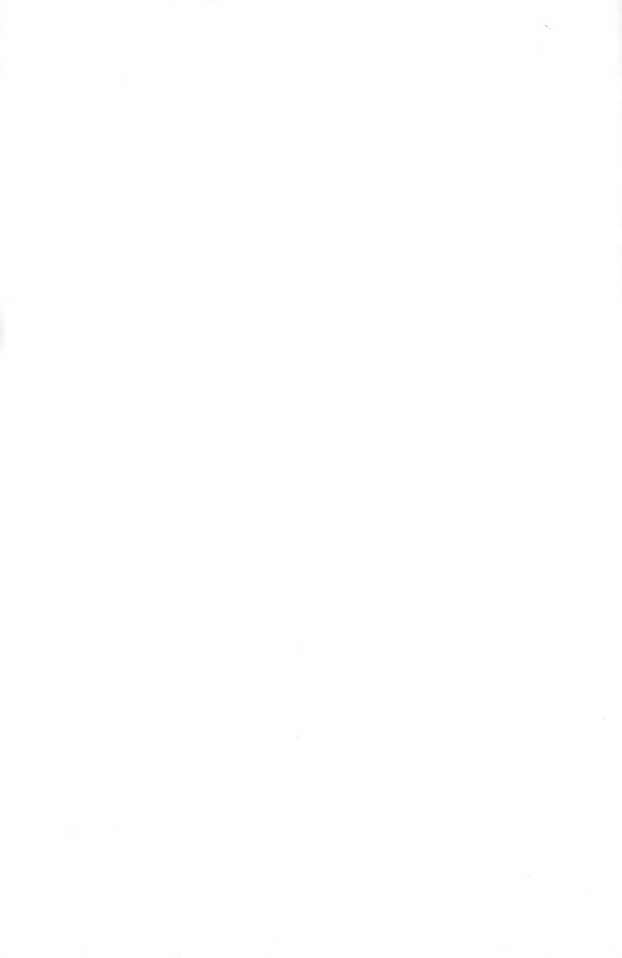

Learning Microbiology and Infectious Diseases: Clinical Case Prep for the USMLE®

Tracey A. H. Taylor, PhD
Associate Professor
Department of Foundational Medical Studies
Oakland University William Beaumont School of Medicine
Rochester, Michigan, USA

Dwayne Baxa, PhD
Assistant Professor
Department of Foundational Medical Studies
Oakland University William Beaumont School of Medicine
Rochester, Michigan, USA

Matthew Sims, MD, PhD
Professor
Department of Internal Medicine
Oakland University William Beaumont School of Medicine
Rochester, Michigan, USA

49 illustrations

Thieme
New York • Stuttgart • Delhi • Rio de Janeiro

Library of Congress Cataloging-in-Publication Data is available from the publisher

Important note: Medicine is an ever-changing science undergoing continual development. Research and clinical experience are continually expanding our knowledge, in particular our knowledge of proper treatment and drug therapy. Insofar as this book mentions any dosage or application, readers may rest assured that the authors, editors, and publishers have made every effort to ensure that such references are in accordance with **the state of knowledge at the time of production of the book.**

Nevertheless, this does not involve, imply, or express any guarantee or responsibility on the part of the publishers in respect to any dosage instructions and forms of applications stated in the book. **Every user is requested to examine carefully** the manufacturers' leaflets accompanying each drug and to check, if necessary in consultation with a physician or specialist, whether the dosage schedules mentioned therein or the contraindications stated by the manufacturers differ from the statements made in the present book. Such examination is particularly important with drugs that are either rarely used or have been newly released on the market. Every dosage schedule or every form of application used is entirely at the user's own risk and responsibility. The authors and publishers request every user to report to the publishers any discrepancies or inaccuracies noticed. If errors in this work are found after publication, errata will be posted at www.thieme.com on the product description page.

Some of the product names, patents, and registered designs referred to in this book are in fact registered trademarks or proprietary names even though specific reference to this fact is not always made in the text. Therefore, the appearance of a name without designation as proprietary is not to be construed as a representation by the publisher that it is in the public domain.

©2020. Thieme. All rights reserved.

Thieme Publishers New York
333 Seventh Avenue, New York, NY 10001 USA
+1 800 782 3488, customerservice@thieme.com

Georg Thieme Verlag KG
Rüdigerstrasse 14, 70469 Stuttgart, Germany
+49 [0]711 8931 421, customerservice@thieme.de

Thieme Publishers Delhi
A-12, Second Floor, Sector-2, Noida-201301
Uttar Pradesh, India
+91 120 45 566 00, customerservice@thieme.in

Thieme Publishers Rio de Janeiro,
Thieme Publicações Ltda.
Edifício Rodolpho de Paoli, 25° andar
Av. Nilo Peçanha, 50 – Sala 2508,
Rio de Janeiro 20020-906 Brasil
+55 21 3172-2297

Cover design: Thieme Publishing Group
Typesetting by Thomson Digital, India

Printed in USA by King Printing Company, Inc.   54321

ISBN 978-1-62623-508-3

Also available as an e-book:
eISBN 978-1-62623-509-0

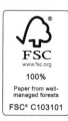

FSC
www.fsc.org
100%
Paper from well-managed forests
FSC® C103101

Contents

Preface

This book is an assortment of clinical cases intended to advance the learning of microbiology and infectious diseases using case studies. Working with cases is the most ideal approach to involve students in the learning process because:

- Every case shows a genuine circumstance, very close to those seen in everyday practice.
- Every case can elicit several problems that must be understood and solved. In other words, it is a problem-based learning process.
- Every case not only requires the knowledge of several disciplines but also the proper utilization of the knowledge to explicit clinical circumstances.

In terms of the organization of the cases, we purposefully intermingled bacteriology, virology, mycology, and parasitology cases in this book, as well as organ systems. We feel that students will gain a better understanding of the topics when they consider all types of organisms for each case, as will be the case when they are considering the diagnosis of real patients. The format of each case is as follows:

- Each case provides relevant clinical information; presenting symptoms and relevant duration, relevant medical history (which may include vaccinations), relevant family history, relevant recent travel, physical examination findings, and lab findings.
- Images are used to support the cases. Images include microscopic images such as Gram stains, electron micrographs, wet mounts, and acid-fast stains, as well as clinical images and skin rashes or lesions.
- Each case is followed by a series of five multiple-choice questions.
  - In most cases, the first question requires the student to identify the most likely causative agent.
  - Other questions address the knowledge of microbiology and infectious diseases that the student needs to assess the case. For example, prevention and precaution measures, transmission, mechanism of action of pathogenesis, diagnostic methods, possible complications, etc.
  - The last question is often related to the pharmacotherapy of the disease.

The questions are designed to prepare students for the United States Medical Licensing Examination (USMLE) and/or Comprehensive Osteopathic Medical Licensing Examination (COMLEX) of the United States Step 1 and Step 2. Five choices are provided for every question, but for each question there is only one best answer.

For each question, answers and explanations are provided on a separate page. This allows students to self-test the entire series of questions before revealing the answers and explanations so that they may completely work through the case and receive optimal formative feedback. The explanations include both the reasons why a given answer is correct and why the distractors are wrong. Many questions are related to the higher levels of Bloom's taxonomy (e.g., analyzing, applying, or evaluating) rather than being simple recall questions.

For each case, keywords are provided so that students may search for a particular area of interest.

Lastly, we have provided a bibliography section for the students. Students are invited to use those references in case they discover that they require a deeper understanding of the material or if they become inspired to seek additional information.

The rationale for this book is related to the current trends in medical education. Now, it is evident that the mere retention of information provided by books is insufficient for meaningful learning. The utilization of information is progressively significant. A vast array of medical problems is available in the literature today, but there are few clinical case books related to microbiology and infectious disease. This book links clinical cases to the application of basic knowledge of microbiology, as well as explains the reasons for using specific drugs in real infectious disease problems, with the goal of promoting critical thinking.

The main audience of the book is medical school students. This book will aid these students in their medical school course work, as well as in preparation for the USMLE and/or COMLEX Step 1 exam. Medical students in years 3 and 4 may also find these cases to be helpful when preparing for the USMLE and/or COMLEX Step 2 exams, shelf exams, and for their clinical rotation coursework. In addition, this book is also useful for students in other medical professions education, including physician assistant students, nursing students, and pharmacy students.

Clinical medicine is a fast-evolving discipline. The authors have referred to reliable sources in order to provide information in accordance with currently accepted standards. However, the authors are aware that in several instances, the information may be controversial. We have tried, as much as possible, to avoid questions addressing controversial issues.

This book is meant to be a companion to the Thieme microbiology question book, thereby giving students more than one option for learning and studying microbiology. This book is not intended to be a substitute for microbiology textbooks. Students are strongly advised to consult their textbooks of microbiology for more in-depth coverage of the subject matter.

Tracey A. H. Taylor, PhD
Dwayne Baxa, PhD
Matthew Sims, MD, PhD

Case 1

Adult with a Cough of a Long Duration

A 36-year-old male presents to his primary care physician with a cough of 4 weeks duration. The cough is paroxysmal, and he sometimes vomits after coughing. Two other people with whom he works have a similar cough. The patient works at a local automobile assembly plant; he is married with a 2-year-old child; and he has no history of cigarette smoking.

On physical examination, the patient initially appears in no acute distress, then experiences a severe coughing attack, which leaves him weak and out of breath. Examination of the head, eyes, ears, nose, and throat (HEENT) revealed a small conjunctival hemorrhage on the left, and several petechiae were noted on the face. Lungs were clear to auscultation. The remainder of the physical examination was benign.

Laboratory studies were obtained, and the complete blood count (CBC) with differential showed a white blood cell (WBC) count of 8,000/ul with a normal differential. Posterior–anterior (PA) and lateral chest X-rays were also obtained and found to be normal.

The physician obtains a nasopharyngeal aspirate that was sent to the microbiology laboratory for Gram stain and culture. An organism not typical for oral-pharyngeal flora and presumed to be the causative pathogen grew on Regan–Lowe agar after overnight incubation at 37°C. The Gram stain is shown in the following figure. A confirmatory direct fluorescent antibody (DFA) staining of the organism isolated from the aspirate was also positive.

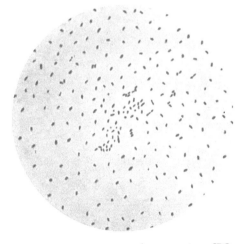

Image courtesy: CDC

Questions

1. Which of the following organisms is the most likely causative agent?

A. *Bordetella pertussis*
B. *Haemophilus influenzae*
C. *Klebsiella pneumoniae*
D. *Legionella pneumophila*
E. *Pseudomonas aeruginosa*

2. How was this infection most likely acquired?

A. Aerosol person to person
B. Arthropod bite
C. Ingestion of food
D. Ingestion of water
E. Sexual transmission

3. For the most likely causative agent, which of the following best describes the pathogenic mechanism leading to the clinical symptoms?

A. Activation of adenylate cyclase by disabling Gi
B. Cleavage of circulating immunoglobulin A (IgA)
C. Inactivation of the 60S ribosome by cleavage of ribosomal RNA (rRNA)
D. Inactivation of host elongation factor 2
E. Prevention of the release of inhibitory neurotransmitter

4. Which of the following best describes the vaccine currently available for prevention of this infection?

A. DNA vaccine
B. Killed whole cell vaccine
C. Live attenuated vaccine
D. Recombinant vector vaccine
E. Subunit vaccine

5. The physician recommends a 5-day course of azithromycin, and the patient takes it appropriately. He returns to the office after completing the course of therapy complaining that his cough is unchanged. Which of the following is the best explanation that the physician can give for the lack of resolution of the cough?

A. Azithromycin is not expected to clear this infection, but it was given because patients expect an antibiotic
B. Coinfection with a second organism is common in this disease, and it is likely that administration of a second antibiotic is warranted
C. It is likely that the infection was resistant to azithromycin, and therapy will need to be altered
D. The purpose of the antibiotic was not to treat the symptoms of the disease but to reduce transmission of the organism
E. The standard dose of azithromycin was too low for this patient's disease, and the dose will need to be doubled

Answers and Explanations

1. Correct: *Bordetella pertussis* (A)

This case describes whooping cough, or *Bordetella pertussis* infection. *B. pertussis* is a fastidious gram-negative coccobacillus that primarily infects children and unvaccinated susceptible individuals. The presentation of pertussis is separated into three stages: the catarrhal phase, which appears as a typical upper respiratory tract infection; the paroxysmal phase, which presents with intense coughing jags and frequently the classic whooping sound of inspiration against a partially closed airway, post-tussive emesis is often seen; and the convalescent phase, which has a chronic cough that can last for weeks. In adults, particularly those who were previously immunized, the classic symptoms such as coughing paroxysms, the whooping sound, and post-tussive emesis may not be seen. The presence of the classic symptoms typically indicates an unvaccinated or undervaccinated individual. In children, a high WBC count (often > 20,000) is seen with a lymphocytosis frequently over 50%. Seeing a young child with a cough and high WBC with significant lymphocytosis is often a diagnostic clue for pertussis. In adults, however, the elevated WBC is rare, and lymphocytosis is generally not seen.
B *Haemophilus influenzae* is incorrect because infections do not present with a paroxysmal cough, and *H. influenzae* are gram-negative bacilli.
C *Klebsiella pneumoniae* is incorrect because infections do not present with a paroxysmal cough, and *K. pneumoniae* are gram-negative bacilli.
D *Legionella pneumophila* is incorrect because they are rarely able to be visualized by Gram stain, and infections do not present with a paroxysmal cough.
E *Pseudomonas aeruginosa* is incorrect because these infections are more often nosocomial or related to cystic fibrosis, which this patient does not have. Also, *P. aeruginosa* are gram-negative bacilli.

2. Correct: Aerosol person to person (A)

Transmission of *B. pertussis* from person-to-person occurs via aerosolized respiratory droplets. There are no identified animal or environmental reservoirs for this pathogen. Humans are the reservoir for *B. pertussis*. The incubation period is 7 to 10 days on average with a maximum of up to 20 days.
B Arthropod bite is incorrect because pertussis is not vector-borne.
C Ingestion of food is incorrect because pertussis is not food-borne.
D Ingestion of water is incorrect because pertussis is not water-borne.
E Sexual transmission is incorrect because pertussis is not sexually transmitted.

3. Correct: Activation of adenylate cyclase by disabling Gi (A)

The virulence factors produced by *B. pertussis* include adherence to ciliated epithelial cells of the trachea and bronchi via pili and filamentous hemagglutinin, endotoxin, pertussis toxin, hemolysin, adenylate cyclase toxin, and tracheal cytotoxin. Pertussis toxin is an A-B5 exotoxin that is secreted by a type IV secretion system and binds to the G-alpha inhibitory subunit inhibiting signal transduction, resulting in increased cyclic adenosine monophosphate (cAMP) and a subsequent increase in mucus production and death of the host cell. This mechanism of action of the pertussis toxin mimics adenylate cyclase activity.
B Cleavage of circulating IgA is incorrect. The cleavage of IgA by bacterial proteases, such as in the case of *H. influenzae*, results in the impairment of antibody-induced entrapment of microbes in mucus secretions.
C Inactivation of the 60S ribosome by cleavage of rRNA is incorrect. This describes the mechanism of action of Shiga toxin.
D Toxin causing inactivation of host elongation factor 2 is incorrect. This describes the mechanism of action of *P. aeruginosa* exotoxin A.
E Toxin that prevents the release of inhibitory neurotransmitter is incorrect. This describes the mechanism of action of *Clostridium botulinum*.

4.   Correct: Subunit vaccine (E)

Prevention of infection is primarily by routine vaccination of infants, children, and adults. Though it was not mentioned explicitly, the patient was likely either unvaccinated or undervaccinated. Appropriate vaccination may have protected him from infection. The diphtheria, tetanus, and pertussis (DTap) vaccine in full strength is given to infants and children, while the reduced dose tetanus-diphtheria-pertussis (Tdap) vaccine is offered to teens and adults. The current vaccine for pertussis is an acellular subunit vaccine, consisting of inactivated pertussis toxin ± filamentous hemagglutinin (FHA), fimbriae, and pertactin (adhesin). The current vaccine does not give lifelong immunity, and boosting in adults is recommended by the Centers for Disease Control and Prevention (CDC) to help prevent transmission to children.

A DNA vaccine is incorrect. The pertussis vaccine is a subunit vaccine. There are no DNA vaccines approved for use in humans at present.

B Killed whole cell vaccine is incorrect. The pertussis vaccine is a subunit vaccine. An example of a killed whole cell vaccine is the previous pertussis vaccine, which is no longer used in the United States.

C Live attenuated vaccine is incorrect. The pertussis vaccine is a subunit vaccine. Example of a live attenuated vaccine is the MMR, nasal influenza, and chickenpox (varicella).

D Recombinant vector vaccine is incorrect. The pertussis vaccine is a subunit vaccine. There are no recombinant vector vaccines approved for use in humans at present.

5.   Correct: The purpose of the antibiotic was not to treat the symptoms of the disease but to reduce transmission of the organism (D)

Treatment of pertussis is generally supportive, particularly in very young children. Cough suppressants have little impact. Antibiotics generally have no impact on the duration of symptoms, though they may shorten the course and decrease the severity if given early in the catarrhal phase. Since pertussis is rarely diagnosed during the catarrhal phase, the addition of antibiotics is to eradicate the *B. pertussis* from the nasopharynx to reduce the spread of the infection (particularly in this case as this patient lives with a child at home and works in a populated environment). The antibiotic of choice is azithromycin (due to dosing schedule, bioavailability, and low side effect profile). Alternative antibiotics include clarithromycin, erythromycin, and for patients older than 2 months intolerant of macrolides, trimethoprim–sulfamethoxazole (TMP–SMX) is a reasonable alternative. TMP–SMX should be avoided in children younger than 2 months due to risk for kernicterus. Azithromycin and erythromycin are both associated with an increased risk of infantile hypertrophic pyloric stenosis, and it is unclear if such a risk exists for clarithromycin. Neither azithromycin nor clarithromycin is approved by the Food and Drug Administration (FDA) for use in children younger than 6 months. Macrolide resistance is very uncommon, and antibiotic testing is generally not performed.

A Azithromycin is not expected to clear this infection, but it was given because patients expect an antibiotic. This is incorrect because it is never correct to give an antibiotic just because a patient wants it.

B Coinfection with a second organism is common in this disease, and it is likely that administration of a second antibiotic is warranted. This is incorrect because coinfection with a second organism is not common in this disease.

C It is likely that the infection was resistant to azithromycin, and therapy will need to be altered. This is incorrect because azithromycin resistance is not commonly described in pertussis.

E The standard dose of azithromycin was too low for this patient's disease and the dose will need to be doubled. This is incorrect because a standard dose is all that is needed.

Additional Diagnostic Information

Diagnosis of *B. pertussis* infection is by nasopharyngeal swab and culture on Regan–Lowe or Bordet–Gengou agar conducted within the first 2 weeks of coughing, or direct fluorescence antibody detection (again early in infection when larger numbers of viable bacteria are still present). Alternatively, polymerase chain reaction (PCR) testing can be conducted up to 4 weeks after the onset of cough. Serological testing using the complement-dependent cytotoxicity (CDC) assay is useful for diagnosis later in infection usually between 2 and 8 weeks but up to 12 weeks following the onset of cough. Nasopharyngeal specimens collected by Dacron swab must be obtained from the respiratory epithelium of the posterior nasopharynx where bacteria levels will be greater. Nasopharyngeal aspirates if available provide the best specimens for bacterial recovery.

Coinfection with viral respiratory pathogens can occur and may complicate differential diagnosis, particularly in adults. Infection in previously vaccinated or undervaccinated adults can lead to atypical presentation with less severe paroxysmal symptoms leading to misdiagnosis.

Keywords: Pertussis, whooping cough, *Bordetella pertussis*, Regan–Lowe, subunit vaccine, nasopharyngeal, azithromycin

Case 2

Child with a Sore Throat and Red Eyes

A mother brings her 6-year-old daughter to her pediatrician with symptoms of a sore throat and red, tearing eyes. The patient complains of itchy eyes when she woke up that morning. Her symptoms started the previous day, and she missed school today. History reveals that the child's vaccinations are up to date and that she has been previously healthy with no prior hospitalizations. Upon examination, the patient is found to have a temperature of 39°C, blood pressure of 90/70 mmHg, and respiratory rate of 20 breaths/min. She has upper lid edema with slight subconjunctival hemorrhage. Her mother mentions that other classmates were also out sick during the past week with similar symptoms.

Questions

1. What is the most likely condition experienced by this child?

A. Allergic conjunctivitis

B. Gonococcal conjunctivitis

C. Keratoconjunctivitis

D. Pharyngoconjunctivitis

E. Endophthalmitis

2. Given the patient history, what is the most likely etiology?

A. Adenovirus

B. Herpes simplex virus type 1 (HSV-1)

C. *Neisseria gonorrhoeae*

D. *Pseudomonas aeruginosa*

E. *Staphylococcus aureus*

3. What is the most likely mode of transmission by the causative agent in this case?

A. Arthropod transmission

B. Bloodborne transmission

C. Droplet transmission

D. Foodborne transmission

E. Waterborne transmission

4. Which is the best method to detect an outbreak of this agent?

A. Clinical diagnosis

B. Culture with immunofluorescence assay

C. Polymerase chain reaction (PCR)

D. Serology

E. Rapid antigen test

5. Which of the following precautions must be used to prevent the spread of this infection from a patient to a health care worker?

A. Gown and gloves

B. N-95 mask

C. Surgical mask and eye protection

D. No specific precautions

E. Washing the hands with dilute bleach

Answers and Explanations

1. Correct: Pharyngoconjunctivitis (D)

This is a case of typical pharyngoconjunctivitis. It is highly infectious and usually is clinically identified by fever, pharyngitis, with enlarged lymph nodes in addition to conjunctivitis (pink eye). This infection is often observed in children. Because of its contagious nature, outbreaks often occur in schools, daycares, and dormitory settings. Swimming pool transmission has also been reported. The upper respiratory symptoms may precede or follow the ocular manifestations. The ocular symptoms may begin in one eye first with an itchy or gritty feeling and later becoming bilateral.
A Allergic conjunctivitis is incorrect because these conditions are not associated with sore throat.
B Gonococcal conjunctivitis is incorrect because the discharge from the eye is not purulent.
C Keratoconjunctivitis is incorrect because there is no apparent corneal involvement in this case.
E Endophthalmitis is incorrect because there is no apparent aqueous or vitreous involvement. It typically presents with decreasing vision and eye discomfort, neither of which describes this patient's symptoms.

2. Correct: Adenovirus (A)

Adenovirus is the most common viral cause of conjunctivitis, but approximately 30% of all cases are due to a bacterial cause. In young children, it is estimated that 5 to 10% of all febrile illness are caused by adenoviruses. The genome of adenoviruses is composed of double-stranded DNA. Adenoviruses are non-enveloped and have an icosahedron shape (see the following figure). It is common practice to diagnosis adenovirus pharyngoconjunctivitis by clinical presentation. However, definitive laboratory confirmation should be employed in order to best determine if antibiotics should be prescribed. The adenovirus infection is a self-limiting infection and should resolve within 2 weeks. During this period the person is still infectious.

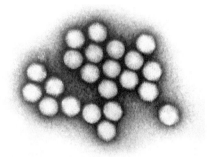

Image courtesy: CDC/ Dr. G. William Gary, Jr.

B HSV-1 is incorrect because it is less likely due to the presence of pharyngitis in this patient. HSV typically causes keratitis, which this patient does not have.
C *Neisseria gonorrhoeae* is incorrect because this patient has no history of risk for *N. gonorrhoeae* infection.
D *Pseudomonas aeruginosa* is incorrect because *P. aeruginosa* more commonly causes nosocomial infections and infections in patients with predisposing factors such as cystic fibrosis.
E *Staphylococcus aureus* is incorrect because eye infections caused by *S. aureus* typically progress rapidly and are characterized by purulent discharge.

3. Correct: Droplet transmission (C)

Adenovirus is a non-enveloped DNA virus and is relatively stable on environmental surfaces, surviving from days to months. Transmission occurs by inhalation of aerosolized droplets as well as fomites generated by hand-to-eye and fecal–oral routes. Transmission has occurred via recreational waters such as swimming pools and spas and is most likely a fecal–oral route, but secretions from eyes or throat can be a possible source. It is not spread via airborne transmission in small particles as is tuberculosis. Adenovirus has 50 serotypes grouped into seven subtypes: A to G. Neutralizing antibodies raised against one subtype do not provide immunity against virus of another subtype allowing for apparent reinfection.

A Arthropod transmission is incorrect because adenovirus is not vector-borne.
B Bloodborne transmission is incorrect because there is no history of blood exposure in this case, and adenovirus is not typically transmitted via the blood.
D Foodborne transmission is incorrect because adenovirus is not food-borne.
E Waterborne transmission is incorrect because while adenovirus can be transmitted through water, transmission was not by this method in this case.

4.   Correct: Polymerase chain reaction (PCR) (C)

All of the listed answers are capable of being utilized in diagnosing pharyngoconjunctivitis. PCR is the best option both for specificity/sensitivity and turn-around-time and is commonly available as part of a respiratory viral panel performed on nasopharyngeal swabs.
A While it is certainly commonplace to diagnose adenovirus by clinical presentation, misdiagnosis is possible and often leads to lack of antibiotic stewardship.
B Cell culture is available for adenovirus detection, and the virus produces a characteristic cytopathic effect visible as cell clumping. However, culture of the virus may take 4 to 7 days for positive confirmation and therefore is rarely used. Shell vial culture (a modified version of traditional cell culture) and immunofluorescent

detection can reduce confirmation to within 3 days.
D Serology testing can detect exposure to adenovirus, but, as most young children are antibody positive by age 5, it has limited utility for diagnosis of acute infection. Serology is not the correct answer.
E There is a point-of-care test that is available for screening adenovirus as a cause of conjunctivitis. However, a negative result does not rule out adenovirus as a cause, and other diagnostic measures should be employed.

5.   Correct: Surgical mask and eye protection (C)

Since adenovirus is spread via droplets which are expelled by coughing, sneezing, or simply talking, the personal protective equipment needed to prevent the spread must include eye protection and a surgical mask.
A Gowns and gloves are not enough to protect from the spread of this virus.
B A N-95 mask would certainly prevent inhalation of adenovirus, but a mask with such a small weave is overkill for adenovirus, and using it without eye protection will not prevent droplets from infecting the health care worker via the conjunctiva.
D, E There is no need to wash with dilute bleach to clean your hands as such measures will not inactivate this non-enveloped virus.

Keywords: Adenovirus, pharyngitis, conjunctivitis, non-enveloped

Case 3

Adult in Respiratory Distress

A 30-year-old construction worker from New Mexico with no significant past medical history was admitted to the hospital with severe shortness of breath. In the emergency room, he stated that he developed a cough in the past few days with fever, muscle aches, nausea, and vomiting. His wife reported that prior to his symptoms he was working overtime, renovating abandoned homes and she initially assumed he was feeling under the weather because he was working so much and not getting enough sleep.

On physical examination his temperature was 38.5°C, blood pressure was 90/50 mmHg, respiratory rate was 28 breaths/min, heart rate was 140 bpm, and oxygen saturation was 75% on room air. A chest X-ray demonstrated bilateral diffuse opacities with Kerley B lines and peribronchial cuffing. His white blood cell count was $26,000 \times 10^9$/L with a predominance of neutrophils and lymphocytes, and noted atypical lymphocytes were observed. The patient's platelet count was 75 with an elevated hematocrit level. A rapid polymerase chain reaction (PCR) test for influenza A is negative. He was admitted into the hospital and given supplemental oxygen but quickly transferred to the intensive care unit and intubated.

Questions

1. Which of the following organisms is the most likely etiology of this infection?

A. Influenza A virus

B. Hantavirus

C. *Legionella pneumophila*

D. *Francisella tularensis*

E. Epstein–Barr virus (EBV)

2. Which of the following is the vector for transmission of the organism?

A. Avian

B. Human

C. Rodent

D. Water

E. Tick

3. Which of the following is the pathogenesis of the patient's pulmonary symptoms?

A. Direct infection of the vascular endothelium of the lungs leading to pulmonary edema

B. Neutrophilic invasion of the lung leading to a multilobar pneumonia

C. Release of toxins into the epithelial lining of the lungs leading to cell death

D. Induction of mucin secretion leading to mucous plugging and obstruction

E. Deposition of secreted proteins along the wall of the alveoli preventing gas exchange

4. Which of the following assays is most often used to detect the causative organism?

A. Culture

B. Enzyme-linked immunosorbent assay (ELISA)

C. Nucleic acid amplification

D. Western blot

E. Gene-chip analysis

5. Which of the following treatments is most appropriate for this patient?

A. Cidofovir

B. Peramivir

C. Acyclovir

D. Doxycycline

E. Supportive care only

Answers and Explanations

This is a case of hantavirus pulmonary syndrome (HPS) caused by genus *Hantavirus* in the *Bunyaviridae* family. Hantaviruses are segmented, negative-stranded RNA viruses. HPS is difficult to distinguish in the initial stages from the other respiratory infections; however, the history of exposure to rodent excreta should be strongly considered in the differential diagnosis. A significant clue in this case is the location of New Mexico, as this is one of the Four Corners states, being New Mexico, Arizona, Colorado, and Utah. This is the region of the first outbreak of HPS in the United States of America in 1993 caused by the viral strain Sin Nombre virus (SNV). Since that time, other cases of HPS caused by other viral strains of hantavirus have been identified in other regions of the United States. The early symptoms of HPS are fatigue, muscle aches, nausea, vomiting, cough, and high fever. These are thought to occur between 1 and 8 weeks after exposure. The late stage of HPS results in shortness of breath caused by the lungs filling with fluid. The virus infects microvascular endothelium resulting in deregulation of fluid accumulation. The fluid increase causes pulmonary edema and cardiac failure. There is 38% mortality in HPS cases.

A While influenza A virus could present with similar symptoms, it is less likely due to the negative rapid PCR test.

C *Legionella pneumophila* can present with similar symptoms but is often associated with exposure to an aerosolized water source such as a cooling tower or air conditioner. In addition, atypical lymphocytes are not normally seen with *Legionella* spp. infection.

D *Francisella tularensis* is not likely because this patient was not exposed to common reservoirs such as rabbits. Pulmonary tularemia frequently presents with nodular infiltrates and pleural effusions.

E EBV is not likely because although this patient has atypical lymphocytes, the other symptoms are not as commonly associated with EBV infection. EBV infection often presents with extreme fatigue.

Hantavirus transmission occurs by inhalation of dried urine, saliva, or feces from infected rodents. The primary host of SNV is the deer mouse (*Peromyscus maniculatus*).

A Hantavirus is not transmitted by birds. There are cases of bird-to-human transmission in the case of the H5N1 influenza A strain.

B Hantavirus is not transmitted by person-to-person contact. Influenza A virus strains are transmitted human-to-human.

D Hantavirus is not transmitted by water. *Legionella* spp. transmission can occur via humidified air originating from a contaminated source.

E Hantavirus is not transmitted by ticks and is not a vector-borne infection.

Hantavirus antigens are primarily found in the endothelium of the capillaries throughout infected patients. Within the lungs this leads to inflammation and endothelial leakage causing pulmonary edema and a variation of acute respiratory distress syndrome.

B Neutrophilic invasion of the lungs is typically seen with bacterial pneumonias.

C Certain bacteria including *Staphylococcus aureus* and *Pseudomonas aeruginosa* produce toxins which can worsen pneumonia but generally are not the primary mode of pathogenesis.

D Mucous plugging can be seen with a number of pulmonary conditions including chronic obstructive pulmonary disease (COPD).

E Buildup of protein along the alveolar walls is the pathogenesis of pulmonary alveolar proteinosis, a rare noninfectious pulmonary syndrome.

4. Correct: Enzyme-linked immunosorbent assay (ELISA) (B)

The detection of *Hantavirus* infection is most often done by serological testing as the viral RNA disappears a few days after symptoms emerge. In the United States of America, the primary tests used are immunoglobulin G (IgG) and IgM ELISAs developed by the Centers for Disease Control and Prevention.

A Cell culture of the virus is difficult due to low viral production and requires biosafety level 3 management, whereas handling of serological specimens can be done under biosafety level 2 conditions.

C Currently, there are not any FDA-approved commercial PCR assays available for *Hantavirus* screening.

D While IgG and IgM can be assayed by Western blot, there is no Western blot available for Hantavirus. These tests use antibody created against recombinant viral N antigen. The viral N antigen is a structural protein that induces a strong antibody response.

E Gene-chip analysis is not available for clinical testing but is strictly used for research.

5. Correct: Supportive care only (E)

Hantavirus has no specific treatment, so the only thing that can be done for a patient with HPS is to provide supportive care including fluids, pressors, oxygen, and mechanical ventilation if needed. Some studies advocate the use of extracorporeal membrane oxygenation and quote survival rates of 66%.

A A cidofovir would be of use for disseminated adenovirus but cidofovir is not of use for treatment of HPS.

B Peramivir would potentially be of use for influenza A but has not been studied in severe cases.

C Acyclovir is used in treating viruses of the herpes family including varicella-zoster virus (VZV) and has been used in the treatment of severe EBV, though the data to support this are mostly based on case reports and meta-analyses.

D Doxycycline can be used to treat atypical pulmonary infections including *Legionella*; it has activity against *Francisella*, and it treats a number of tick-borne illnesses.

Keywords: Pneumonia, Sin Nombre virus, Hantavirus, hemorrhagic fever with renal syndrome, robovirus

Case 4

Adolescent with Sore Throat and Malaise

A 14-year-old female is brought to her primary care physician by her mother. The patient has concerns of a sore throat, headache, fever, and fatigue for the past 24 hours. Her mother states that the patient has had these types of symptoms one or more times per year for the past 5 years and requests some antibiotics. Physical examination reveals a temperature of 38.5°C, cervical lymphadenopathy, and enlarged tonsils. A white exudate and erythematous mucous membranes can be seen upon examination of the throat. A rapid strep test is performed in the office and is negative. A throat swab is obtained and sent for Gram stain and culture. The Gram stain of the throat swab is shown in the figure below. Twenty-four hours later, cultures confirm the diagnosis.

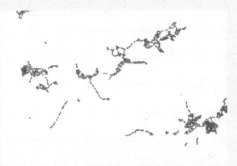

Image courtesy: CDC

Questions

1. Which of the following organisms is the most likely causative agent?

A. Adenovirus

B. Epstein–Barr virus

C. *Haemophilus influenzae* type b

D. *Moraxella catarrhalis*

E. *Streptococcus pyogenes*

2. Which of the following is an important virulence factor of the causative agent?

A. M protein

B. Polyribose-ribitol phosphate capsule

C. Polysaccharide capsule

D. Toxin that inhibits host cell protein synthesis

E. Toxin that stimulates adenylate cyclase

3. Which of the following is a possible complication of this patient's infection if the organism is inadequately treated?

A. Antibiotic-associated colitis

B. Encephalitis

C. Hemolytic uremic syndrome

D. Polyarthritis

E. Rheumatic fever

4. Which of the following best explains why the rapid test result was negative?

A. The rapid test detects patient antibodies

B. The rapid test is less sensitive

C. The sore throat is caused by another organism

D. The result was interpreted incorrectly

E. There were no organisms present

5. Which of the following is the most appropriate treatment for this patient?

A. No antimicrobial treatment, supportive care only

B. Acyclovir

C. Azithromycin

D. Ciprofloxacin

E. Penicillin

Answers and Explanations

1. Correct: *Streptococcus pyogenes* (E)

This case describes a teenager presenting with a likely strep throat infection. The results of the Gram-stained throat swab show gram-positive cocci in chains, which if confirmed as a pathogen would rule out any choices suggesting a viral causative agent (i.e., adenovirus and Epstein–Barr virus); however, Gram stain alone from an oral-pharyngeal swab cannot distinguish this; there are many bacteria in the mouth and throat and many be suggestive of *Streptococcus* spp. based on morphology. In this case, we can apply one of the scoring systems which is used to help determine if strep throat is the likely cause of the patient's illness. A common scoring system is the modified Centor score, in this system one point is given for each of the following: absence of cough, swollen and tender cervical lymph nodes, temperature greater than 38°C, tonsillar swelling or exudates, and age less than 15 (1 point is subtracted for age > 44). The patient does not indicate a runny nose or cough; she has swollen, tender cervical nodes; a fever; tonsillar exudate; and is 14 years old. This gives a Centor score of 5. With 0 point the risk of *Streptococcus pyogenes* pharyngitis is 1 to 2.5%, with 1 point the risk is 5 to 10%, with 2 points the risk is 11 to 17%, with 3 points the risk is 28 to 35%, and with greater than or equal to 4 points the risk is 51 to 53%.

A, B While the patient's symptoms may indicate a viral etiology, the image in the Gram stain shows that it is a bacterial cause.

C *Haemophilus influenzae* type b are gram-negative, which is not seen on the Gram stain. In addition, Hib is less likely than *S. pyogenes* (also known as group A *Streptococcus* or GAS) to cause the described symptoms.

D *Moraxella catarrhalis* are gram-negative rods, which is not seen on the Gram stain and are less likely to cause the symptoms described.

2. Correct: M protein (A)

A major virulence factor of *S. pyogenes* is the M protein, which is a surface protein that protects the organism from phagocytosis. The M protein can be used for serotyping *S. pyogenes* strains as some are more prevalent in rheumatic fever (type 5 M protein). Other *S. pyogenes* virulence factors include streptolysin O, hyaluronidase, streptokinase, nicotinamide adenine dinucleotidase (NADase), and pyrogenic exotoxins. *H. influenzae* has a polyribose-ribitol phosphate capsule.

B, C Some strains of *S. pyogenes* produce a capsule of hyaluronic acid; therefore the answers of polyribose-ribitol phosphate capsule and polysaccharide capsule are incorrect.

D, E *S. pyogenes* pyrogenic exotoxins induce fever and lymphocyte blastogenesis and act as superantigens. They do not inhibit host cell protein synthesis or stimulate adenylate cyclase.

3. Correct: Rheumatic fever (E)

The major complications of *S. pyogenes* infections are acute rheumatic fever and poststreptococcal glomerulonephritis. Rheumatic fever involves molecular mimicry between certain M-protein epitopes and host cardiac tissues. Scarlet fever or scarlatina can also be associated with *S. pyogenes* infections.

A Antibiotic-associated colitis can develop following infection with *Clostridium difficile.*

B Strep throat is not typically associated with postinfectious encephalitis.

C Hemolytic uremic syndrome is a possible complication of an enterohemorrhagic *Escherichia coli* (EHEC) infection.

D Polyarthritis is typically associated with *Campylobacter*, *Salmonella*, and *Shigella* infections and is termed reactive arthritis.

4. Correct: The rapid test is less sensitive (B)

This patient's diagnostic tests are as follows: the rapid test was negative, but the cultures were positive. In children and adolescents, the guidelines state that if the patient's symptoms are suggestive of strep throat, then cultures should be ordered even if the rapid test is negative. The rapid strep test, also called the rapid streptococcal antigen test or RSAT, involves performing a throat swab on the patient, and the test can be processed at the bedside. An enzyme or acid degradation of the pathogen results in the extraction of bacterial antigens from the swab. The presence of the streptococcal antigens can be detected by the test with a specificity of greater than 95% and a sensitivity of 70 to 90%. Throat culture is the gold standard for GAS diagnosis with a sensitivity of 90 to 95%, as such cultures are more sensitive when compared with the rapid test.

A The rapid test detects bacterial antigens and not patient antibodies, therefore that answer is incorrect.

C Given the results of the Gram stain and culture, it is unlikely the sore throat was caused by another organism.

D We can presume that an error was not made in interpreting the results of the rapid test as the interpretation of the rapid streptococcal antigen test (RSAT) is quite simple, especially if positive and negative controls were run in parallel.

E Given the results of the Gram stain and culture (see figure), this sore throat was caused by a bacterial agent.

Keywords: *Streptococcus pyogenes*, strep throat, rapid test, sore throat, rheumatic fever

5.   Correct: Penicillin (E)

According to guidelines, penicillin is still the first choice for the treatment of *S. pyogenes* pharyngitis. The reasons for this choice include proven efficacy and safety, low cost, and a narrow spectrum of activity.

A Even though *S. pyogenes* pharyngitis is a self-limited disease, treatment with appropriate antibiotics is still indicated. The reasons for this are the shortening of symptoms, the elimination of the carriage state, the reduction in peritonsillar abscess, and the reduction in rheumatic fever (which is still a significant problem in developing countries).

B Acyclovir is active against herpes simplex virus (HSV), which is the cause of mononucleosis but in studies has never been shown to have any significant effect on the course of mononucleosis and is not active against strep throat (GAS).

C Azithromycin is a second-line choice for strep throat to be considered in patients with significant allergy to penicillin.

D Ciprofloxacin has no significant activity against *S. pyogenes*.

Case 5

Toddler with Upper Respiratory Symptoms

A 4-year-old girl is brought to her pediatrician by her mother with complaints of cough, rhinorrhea, irritability, and sinus congestion. The mother states that her daughter has been pulling on her right ear, especially when she is laying in bed at night. Past medical history indicates that the child's vaccinations are all up to date. Physical examination reveals a cloudy, bulging eardrum with decreased mobility and a visible meniscus, as well as a low-grade fever. A tympanocentesis is performed, and purulent fluid is recovered and sent to the microbiology laboratory for Gram stain and culture. Gram stain reveals short gram-negative bacilli (see figure below). The next day, there is no growth on blood agar, but gray colonies are seen on chocolate agar after 48 hours.

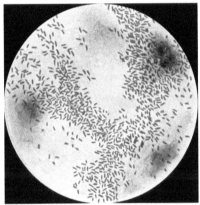

Image courtesy: CDC

Questions

1. Which of the following organisms is the most likely causative agent?

A. *Haemophilus influenzae*

B. *Moraxella catarrhalis*

C. *Neisseria gonorrhoeae*

D. *Streptococcus pneumoniae*

E. *Streptococcus pyogenes*

2. Which of the following best describes the vaccine currently available for prevention of infection by more pathogenic strains of the most likely causative organism?

A. DNA vaccine

B. Killed whole cell vaccine

C. Live attenuated vaccine

D. Recombinant vector vaccine

E. Subunit vaccine

3. How was this infection most likely acquired?

A. Aerosol person to person

B. Arthropod bite

C. Ingestion of food

D. Ingestion of water

E. Sexual transmission

4. Which of the following describes an important virulence factor produced by the most likely causative agent?

A. Exotoxin A

B. Flagella

C. Hyaluronidase

D. Immunoglobulin A (IgA) protease

E. M protein

5. Per guidelines, the patient is initiated on treatment with high-dose amoxicillin. However, 2 days later there is no significant improvement. Which of the following represents the most likely cause of treatment failure and the appropriate next step in treatment?

A. Admit the patient for intravenous ceftriaxone as the failure is likely due to inability to achieve appropriate antibiotic levels with oral medications

B. Change the patient to amoxicillin–clavulanic acid as the frequent dosing of amoxicillin is likely causing the patient to miss doses, and the less frequent dosing schedule for amoxicillin–clavulanic acid will eliminate this problem

C. Change the patient to clindamycin as the organism is likely to be resistant to beta-lactams

D. Change the patient to trimethoprim–sulfamethoxazole (TMP–SMX) since TMP–SMX is the drug of choice for treating the pathogen isolated

E. Change the patient to amoxicillin–clavulanic acid as the most likely cause of failure is presence of a beta-lactamase which would be inhibited by the clavulanic acid

Answers and Explanations

1. Correct: *Haemophilus influenzae* (A)

This describes an otitis media infection. The most common causative organisms for otitis media in a child over the age of 6 weeks are *Streptococcus pneumoniae, Haemophilus influenzae,* and *Moraxella catarrhalis. S. pneumoniae* are gram-positive cocci while *M. catarrhalis* are gram-negative coccobacilli or diplococci, so the most likely agent based on the Gram stain morphology is *H. influenzae.* Furthermore, *H. influenzae* does not grow on blood agar, as described in the case.

B This option is incorrect because *M. catarrhalis* are gram-negative coccobacilii or diplococci while gram-negative bacilli can be seen in the image.

C This option is incorrect because *N. gonorrhoeae* are gram-negative cocci and more commonly diplococci while gram-negative bacilli can be seen in the image.

D This option is incorrect because *S. pneumoniae* are gram-positive cocci while gram-negative bacilli can be seen in the image.

E This option is incorrect because *S. pyogenes* are gram-positive cocci while gram-negative bacilli can be seen in the image.

2. Correct: Subunit vaccine (E)

The *H. influenzae* type b vaccine, or Hib, was developed for the prevention of epiglottitis and meningitis, also caused by this organism. The vaccine is composed of the polyribose-ribitol phosphate (PRP) capsular antigen of the type b capsule. It is a subunit vaccine as only a portion of the organisms antigens is present in the vaccine. PRP is a major virulence factor of the type b strain. It is notable that in this case the patient has been vaccinated, so it can be assumed that an unencapsulated strain of *H. influenzae* is causing the infection. Immunization with Hib does not confer cross-protection against the nonencapsulated strains of the organism.

A DNA vaccine is incorrect. There are no DNA vaccines approved for use in humans at present.

B Killed whole cell vaccine is incorrect. Example of a killed whole cell vaccine is the previous pertussis vaccine which is no longer used in the United States.

C Live attenuated vaccine is incorrect. Examples of a live attenuated vaccine include the MMR, nasal influenza, and chickenpox (varicella) vaccines.

D Recombinant vector vaccine is incorrect. There are no recombinant vector vaccines approved for use in humans at present.

3. Correct: Aerosol person to person (A)

Because humans are believed to be the natural host for *H. influenzae,* this infection was most likely transmitted via person-to-person by respiratory droplets. It is mentioned in the case that the patient also displays cold-like symptoms, indicating that the patient may be coinfected with an upper respiratory tract infection (also commonly transmitted by respiratory droplets).

B Arthropod transmission is incorrect because *H. influenzae* is not vector-borne.

C Foodborne transmission is incorrect because *H. influenzae* is not food-borne.

D Waterborne transmission is incorrect because *H. influenzae* is not water-borne.

E Sexual transmission is incorrect because *H. influenzae* is not sexually transmitted.

4. Correct: Immunoglobulin A (IgA) protease (D)

Many nonencapsulated strains of *H. influenzae* produce IgA protease. Recall that IgA is important for host defense of mucosal surfaces, therefore many pathogens that infect mucosal surfaces are able to produce a protease that can actively break down this immunoglobulin. *H. influenzae* produces at least three types of IgA proteases that cleave different regions of the IgA1 hinge.

A Exotoxin A is a virulence factor of *Pseudomonas aeruginosa* that ADP-ribosylates elongation factor 2, and therefore halts host cell protein synthesis.

B Flagella are produced by motile bacteria, but *H. influenzae* are nonmotile and therefore do not produce flagella.

C Hyaluronidases are produced by many streptococcal species and are important virulence factors during infection to enable pathogens to hydrolyze hyaluronic acid and facilitate organism spread along fascial planes.

E Finally, the M protein is an important virulence factor for *Streptococcus pyogenes* infections and is used for strain typing.

5.   Correct: Change the patient to amoxicillin–clavulanic acid as the most likely cause of failure is presence of a beta-lactamase which would be inhibited by the clavulanic acid (E)

In this case, the most likely cause of *H. influenzae* not responding to amoxicillin is the production of a beta-lactamase, which accounts for greater than 90% of resistance to amoxicillin in *H. influenzae*.

A Oral antibiotics are considered adequate for nonsevere acute otitis media.

B The guidelines recommend that in cases of amoxicillin failure, amoxicillin-clavulanic acid should be used. However, both amoxicillin and amoxicillin-clavulanic acid are given at the same dosing schedule of twice a day and should achieve appropriate levels for acute otitis media.

C Changing to clindamycin is not appropriate because clindamycin is not active against gram negative bacteria.

D TMP-SMX is not the drug of choice for *H. influenzae* and is not in the guidelines for treatment.

Additional Diagnostic Information

There are numerous reasons a patient can fail treatment with an antibiotic. There are three main categories: (1) the antibiotic is not active against the bacteria, (2) the antibiotic is not reaching the bacteria, and (3) bacteria are not present. Reasons that an antibiotic may not be active against a bacterial infection are: (1) incorrect assumption on the identity of the bacteria, thus using the wrong antibiotic, or (2) the existence of antibiotic resistance. Reasons that an antibiotic may fail to reach the bacteria include the bacterial infection being in a protected space such as in the central nervous system where antibiotics may not penetrate due to the blood–brain barrier, too low a dose of antibiotic or too infrequent a dose of antibiotic thus not enough antibiotic is reaching the bacteria, or inactivation of the antibiotic before it gets to the bacteria due to pH or other inhibitors (e.g., surfactant in the lungs inactivating daptomycin due to calcium sequestration). Not treating a bacterial infection includes diseases which mimic infections such as cancer, autoimmune diseases, and connective tissue disorders, diseases which are sequelae of infections such as poststreptococcal glomerulonephritis, and infections which have progressed past the point of no return such as end-stage septic shock from disseminated meningococcemia.

Keywords: Otitis media, ear infection, *Haemophilus influenzae*, chocolate agar, Hib vaccine

Case 6

Elderly Male with Two Days of Fever, Chills, and Cough

A 69-year-old male presents to the emergency department with complaints of fever, chills, and cough for the past 48 hours which his wife says is getting worse. Past medical history reveals that he is a smoker who has smoked one pack of cigarettes a day for the past 50 years and that he has no recent hospitalizations or illnesses. The patient's wife reports that he is frequently coughing up brown-colored sputum in the mornings but that the character of the sputum has recently changed. He is a retired automobile mechanic and he enjoys camping. No one else in his family has similar symptoms and his wife reports he has had no sick contacts. She also states that he has no allergies. Physical examination reveals a slightly confused man with a temperature of 38.9°C, blood pressure of 130/90 mmHg, a pulse of 105 bpm, a respiratory rate of 32 breaths/min, and an oxygen saturation of 92% on room air. A radiograph shows slightly hyperinflated lungs and scattered bullae as well as an infiltrate that is localized to the right lower lobe. A sputum sample is obtained for Gram stain and is shown in the figure below.

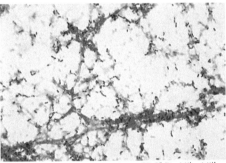

Image courtesy: CDC/ Dr. Mike Miller

Questions

1. Which of the following organisms is the most likely causative agent?

A. *Chlamydia psittaci*

B. *Legionella pneumophila*

C. *Pneumocystis jiroveci*

D. *Staphylococcus aureus*

E. *Streptococcus pneumonia*

2. In terms of hemolysis and optochin, which of the following best describes the laboratory test results that would be expected if the causative agent was cultured and tested?

A. Alpha hemolysis, optochin sensitive

B. Alpha hemolysis, optochin resistant

C. Beta hemolysis, optochin sensitive

D. Beta hemolysis, optochin resistant

E. Gamma hemolysis, optochin sensitive

F. Gamma hemolysis, optochin resistant

3. A commonly available antigen test can potentially confirm the diagnosis by testing which of the following patient samples?

A. Blood

B. Saliva

C. Stool

D. Sweat

E. Urine

4. Which of the following best describes the vaccine available for control and prevention of infections by the causative agent?

A. DNA vaccine

B. Conjugate vaccine

C. Live attenuated vaccine

D. Toxoid vaccine

E. Whole cell heat-killed vaccine

5. Which of the following antibiotic treatments would be most appropriate to start in this patient?

A. Penicillin G

B. Azithromycin

C. Vancomycin

D. Piperacillin–tazobactam

E. Ceftriaxone

Answers and Explanations

1. Correct: *Streptococcus pneumonia* (E)

Streptococcus pneumoniae is the most common cause of lobar pneumonia. Rust-colored/brown sputum is also common for *S. pneumoniae* infections. Furthermore, the Gram stain of the sputum shows gram-positive cocci in pairs with a nonstaining halo (indicative of the capsule), which is the characteristic cellular morphology for *S. pneumoniae*.

A *Chlamydia psittaci* could be possible because this patient enjoys the outdoors, so he does have possible exposure to birds and bird droppings; however, the Gram stain of the sputum is suggestive of gram-positive cocci, and *C. psittaci* are non-Gram staining.

B Because of the advanced age of the patient in this case, *Legionella pneumophila* should be considered. However, because the onset is acute and not subacute, and *L. pneumophila* do not Gram stain well and are gram-negative, this is not the most likely causative agent.

C *Pneumocystis jiroveci* would be a possible causative agent if the patient was HIV positive or immunocompromised, but that is not the case.

D *Staphylococcus aureus* would be more likely if the patient had a recent history of an influenza infection or was an intravenous drug user.

2. Correct: Alpha hemolysis, optochin sensitive (A)

S. pneumoniae are alpha hemolytic, meaning that the organisms have the ability to partially lyse the red blood cells on blood agar plates when grown in culture. These organisms are characteristically inhibited by optochin and therefore are unable to grow (i.e., are sensitive to) in the presence of optochin on laboratory agar plates. *S. pneumoniae* are also characteristically lysed by bile salts (deoxycholate) due to the presence of an autolytic enzyme.

B *S. pneumoniae* is alpha hemolytic but they are sensitive to optochin. Viridans group *Streptococcus* are alpha hemolytic and are optochin resistant.

C *S. pyogenes* is beta hemolytic but is optochin resistant and is not the causative agent in this case.

D *S. pyogenes* is beta hemolytic and is optochin resistant but is not the most likely causative agent in this case.

E The former Group D *Streptococcus* have been reclassified as *Enterococcus* spp. and are gamma hemolytic and are not the causative agent in this case.

F *Enterococcus* spp. are gamma hemolytic, optochin resistant, and are not the causative agent in this case.

3. Correct: Urine (E)

The pneumococcal urinary antigen test is an assay that detects *S. pneumoniae* cell wall antigens from patient urine. As such, it is noninvasive and does not require the patient to provide sputum. This test was developed to fill the need to a speedy and accurate diagnosis of pneumonia. The test is approximately 70 to 90% sensitive and 80 to 100% specific in adults. Cell culture from sputum sample is the gold standard for diagnosis, but it requires the patient to generate sputum, and results take at least 24 to 48 hours. Polymerase chain reaction (PCR) of pleural fluid will also yield a definitive diagnosis, but obtaining pleural fluid is more invasive, and the results will take longer than for a urine antigen test. A throat swab rapid test is used to presumptively diagnose *S. pyogenes* or strep throat.

A, B, C, D Other bodily fluids cannot be used for this rapid test. There is no rapid antigen test available for blood, saliva, stool, or sweat.

4. Correct: Conjugate vaccine (B)

Two different types of vaccines for *S. pneumoniae* are approved for use in the United States. The pneumococcal polysaccharide vaccine (PPSV) contains capsular polysaccharides and is used for routine vaccination

25

in selected adults and children younger than 2 years. PPSV is not used for infants because polysaccharide antigens do not illicit a strong immune response. The second vaccine is the pneumococcal conjugate vaccine (PCV). The polysaccharide antigens are covalently linked to a protein carrier in order to increase the immunogenicity of this vaccine. As a result, PCV is used for routine vaccination of infants and toddlers as well as adults older than 65 years.

A At present, there are no DNA vaccines for routine vaccination for humans.

C Examples of live attenuated vaccines include vaccines against rotavirus, varicella, MMR, and the nasal spray vaccine for influenza (FluMist).

D An example of a toxoid vaccine is the tetanus vaccine (*Clostridium tetani*).

E Examples of inactivated (whole cell heat-killed) vaccines include the polio vaccine (Salk), the injected influenza vaccine, and the pertussis vaccine (*Bordetella pertussis*).

5.   Correct: Ceftriaxone (E)

All of the listed choices potentially have activity against *S. pneumoniae*. Ceftriaxone is active against *S. pneumoniae* and penicillin-resistant *S. pneumoniae* and is an appropriate first-line antibiotic for the treatment of *S. pneumoniae*.

A According to current guidelines, when the etiologic agent is established or strongly suspected, it is reasonable to switch from an empiric therapy to a more directed therapy. At this point, no sensitivity data are known to determine whether the *S. pneumoniae* in this case is penicillin-resistant or not. As such penicillin is not a reasonable choice.

B Azithromycin is reasonable for simple community-acquired pneumonia (CAP) where there is no suspected resistance, but this patient is somewhat more complicated with underlying chronic obstructive pulmonary disease (COPD), and his CURB-65 score is at least 3 with confusion, respirations greater than or equal to 30 breaths/min, and age greater than or equal to 65. No data are given for uremia, and his blood pressure is not less than 90 systolic or 60 diastolic. As such, azithromycin is not a reasonable choice as a single agent.

C Vancomycin would be appropriate if he had a high-grade allergy to beta-lactams and suspicion for penicillin-resistant *S. pneumoniae*; as he has no allergies, vancomycin is not an appropriate choice.

D Piperacillin–tazobactam is appropriate for hospital-acquired pneumonia (HAP) or health care-associated pneumonia (HCAP) but not for CAP where there is low suspicion for gram-negative pathogens, particularly *Pseudomonas aeruginosa*.

Keywords: *Streptococcus pneumoniae*, pneumonia, sputum, hemolysis, pneumococcal vaccine, ceftriaxone

Case 7 | Severely Ill Elderly Male in Respiratory Distress

A 71-year-old male with mild chronic obstructive pulmonary disease (COPD) is brought to the emergency department by his daughter with symptoms of a high fever, chest pain, shortness of breath, and a nonproductive cough. He claims that the fever and a headache started 3 days before. Upon examination, his temperature is found to be 104°F and oxygen saturation at 82% on room air. The patient was tachycardic at 119 bpm. Coarse breathing sounds were heard on auscultation. The patient is not fully responsive. The daughter is asked about his medical history and states that other than the mild COPD, which he only uses some inhalers for, he is very healthy and hasn't been hospitalized in years. He hasn't traveled and has no sick contacts or animal exposures. He recently moved in with his daughter and her family. Since it is the summer and the weather is good, he states that he spends most of his time during the day (when the children are at school) in the garden area of their apartment complex sitting by the fountain and reading. He is up to date on his immunizations and received PPSV23 and PCV13 as well as herpes zoster vaccination and a booster for pertussis since he is around his grandchildren all the time now.

A chest radiograph showed pleural effusions and confluent infiltrates in the left lower lobe. A bronchoalveolar lavage (BAL) was conducted. Gram stain of the specimen did not detect any organisms. Culture of the BAL specimen demonstrated growth on buffered charcoal yeast extract agar but not 5% sheep blood agar. A Gram stain from the culture is shown in the figure below.

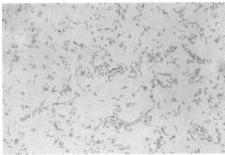

Image courtesy: CDC/ Dr. Gilda Jones

Questions

1. Based on the patient history and laboratory findings, what is the most likely cause of this patient's symptoms?

A. *Influenza virus*

B. *Legionella pneumophila*

C. *Mycobacterium tuberculosis*

D. *Pneumocystis jirovecii*

E. *Streptococcus pneumoniae*

2. In addition to culture, which of the following is the preferred method for diagnosis?

A. Direct fluorescent antibody stain of lung biopsy

B. Paired serology

C. Polymerase chain reaction (PCR)

D. Sputum Gram stain

E. Urinary antigen test

3. What is the most likely transmission scenario for this illness?

A. Casual contact

B. Contaminated vaccine

C. Food contamination

D. Sexual transmission

E. Water droplets

4. This organism has multiple life stages. Which of the following best describes its life cycle characteristics?

A. Facultative anaerobe

B. Facultative capnophile

C. Facultative intracellular

D. Facultative spore forming

E. Facultative thermophile

5. Of the following, which is the most active therapeutic agent for this patient's infection?

A. Azithromycin

B. Ceftriaxone

C. Isoniazid

D. Oseltamivir

E. Trimethoprim–sulfamethoxazole

Answers and Explanations

1. Correct: *Legionella pneumophila* (B)

This is a case of pneumonia caused by *Legionella pneumophila*. *Legionella* spp. exist in freshwater environments and can inhabit artificial water systems where proper disinfection is lacking and transmission to humans is more likely to occur. Individuals at greatest risk for infection are those with chronic lung disease, smokers, those with weak immune systems, and people older than 50 years (such as the patient in this case). *Legionella* spp. were initially identified as a result of an outbreak of pneumonia in 1976 at a convention of the American Legion in Philadelphia, owning to its name. A related illness also attributed to *Legionella* is known as Pontiac fever and was first identified in Pontiac, Michigan. This illness does not result in pneumonia and is less severe in its manifestations. Symptoms include fever and muscle aches and usually last about a week after initial signs.
A Influenza virus is not the correct answer because of the symptoms described and also because gram-negative bacilli can be seen from the Gram stain, indicating a bacterial cause rather than viral.
C *Mycobacterium tuberculosis* is incorrect because this patient's symptoms are not typical of the clinical presentation of tuberculosis, and also *M. tuberculosis* does not stain by the Gram's method.
D *Pneumocystis jirovecii* is incorrect as this patient would unlikely be infected with *Pneumocystis carinii* pneumonia (PCP) due to the lack of a diagnosis of HIV infection.
E While *Streptococcus pneumoniae* is the most common cause of community-acquired pneumonia; they are gram-positive cocci, whereas gram-negative bacilli are seen in the figure.

2. Correct: Urinary antigen test (E)

L. pneumophila are difficult to culture. *Legionella* spp. have complex nutritional requirements and do not grow on standard blood plates. Agars based on buffered charcoal yeast extract (BCYE) medium containing cysteine, high concentrations of iron and activated charcoal are the usual medium of choice for culture. The most commonly used laboratory test for diagnosis is the urinary antigen test. However, this test only detects antigen for serogroup 1, which is the most common cause of legionellosis. There are 42 *Legionella* species with 64 serogroups capable of causing human disease. Because of this diversity, culture is used as a confirmatory test when urine antigen tests are negative.
A A direct fluorescent antibody (DFA) stain of lung biopsy can be used for diagnosis but is not routine due to the invasiveness of this procedure.
B Paired serology is not common for the diagnosis of *Legionella* spp. infection.
C There are currently no Food and Drug Administration (FDA) approved PCR assays available, and routine PCR-based tests are not available at every hospital center.
D Sputum Gram stain is not typically used for diagnosis because *Legionella* spp. are difficult to Gram stain, so a negative Gram stain is common with *Legionella* spp. infection.

3. Correct: Water droplets (E)

Legionella spp. survive in warm water environments where improper disinfection occurs, or they can survive intracellularly in amoeba, which are not routinely killed by chlorination. Sources such as shower heads, water cooling systems, hot tubs and spas, and water features have all been documented to be a source of the bacteria. Transmission to humans occurs when aerosolized water droplets are inhaled.
A Casual contact is incorrect because of dose transmission (there would not be enough *Legionella* transmitted to cause an infection).
B Contaminated vaccine is incorrect because there is no vaccine for *Legionella* infection.
C Food contamination is incorrect because *Legionella* is not food-borne.
D Sexual transmission is incorrect because *Legionella* is not a sexually transmitted infection.

4. Correct: Facultative intracellular (C)

Legionella spp. are unlike other bacterial pneumonia pathogens, in that they do not reside within the upper respiratory tract (i.e., these bacteria are not normal flora) but infect alveolar macrophages and alveolar epithelial cells as intracellular organisms. In the natural environment, *Legionella* spp. are intracellular pathogens of amoeba. In all instances, cells take up the bacteria via phagocytic processes. *Legionella* spp. are facultative intracellular because they are also able to survive and grow outside of eukaryotic host cells. Once internalized, the bacteria are able to evade phagolysosomal degradation. While *Legionella* spp. can be cultured on artificial media, they are only pathogenic when they complete an intracellular life cycle.

A *Legionella* spp. are aerobic organisms, not anaerobic.

B *Legionella* spp. are not capnophilic (capnophiles thrive in the presence of high concentrations of carbon dioxide).

D *Legionella* spp. are not able to form spores.

E *Legionella* spp. cannot survive at elevated temperatures and are, therefore, not thermophiles.

5. Correct: Azithromycin (A)

The two most appropriate therapies for *L. pneumophila* infections are macrolides, such as azithromycin, or respiratory quinolones, such as levofloxacin.

B Ceftriaxone is the most appropriate treatment for *S. pneumoniae* (the most common causative agent of community-acquired pneumonia), and it is likely this patient will receive both ceftriaxone and azithromycin as per the guidelines for the treatment of community-acquired pneumonia.

C Isoniazid would be part of a regimen for tuberculosis (TB) but would only be given alone for latent TB infection.

D Oseltamivir would be given for suspicion of influenza virus which is unlikely in the summer months.

E Trimethoprim–sulfamethoxazole would be the first-line treatment for PCP but has no activity against *Legionella* spp.

Keywords: *Legionella pneumophila*, atypical pneumonia, waterborne, COPD

Case 8

Teenager with a Two-Week-Long Cough

A 16-year-old adolescent female presents to her primary care physician with a cough of 2-weeks duration. No one else in her household has a similar cough. She is a student and has no history of cigarette smoking. Her past medical history is remarkable for recurrent lung infections that have been relatively mild; she has never been admitted to the hospital for treatment of one of her infections before. She states that this cough is much worse than her "usual" cough or any of the prior infections. She has a previous confirmed molecular genetic laboratory test finding of being heterozygous with a delta F508 mutation in the cystic fibrosis transmembrane conductance regulator *(CFTR)* gene.

Physical examination reveals a temperature of 38.7°C, a heart rate of 120 bpm, and a respiratory rate of 30 breaths/min; she is markedly dyspneic, has a reduced forced vital capacity (FVC), and the cough is productive of greenish sputum. Her oxygen saturation is found to be 82% while her baseline oxygen saturation is 95%.

Laboratory studies were obtained, and the complete blood count (CBC) with differential showed white blood cell (WBC) count 18.5×10^9 cells/L with a marked left shift. Posteroanterior (PA) and lateral chest X-rays were also obtained and showed hyperinflation and bronchiectasis and "tram tracks" in the upper lobes. There is a dense consolidation with air bronchograms involving most of the left lung.

The physician obtains a sample of the sputum that is sent to the microbiology laboratory for Gram stain and culture. A Gram stain is shown in the figure below. The predominant organism grew as mucoid colonies on blood agar at 37°C after 24 hours with beta hemolysis and a metallic sheen. The organism is citrate positive and oxidase positive.

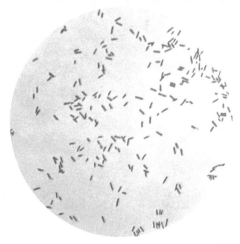

Image courtesy: CDC

Questions

1. Which of the following organisms is the most likely causative agent?

A. *Legionella pneumophila*

B. *Mycoplasma pneumoniae*

C. *Pseudomonas aeruginosa*

D. *Staphylococcus aureus*

E. *Streptococcus pneumonia*

2. Which of the following would best describe the growth of the most likely causative agent on MacConkey agar?

A. Growth with clearing around each colony

B. Growth with colorless colonies

C. Growth with pink colonies

D. No growth

E. Swarming growth

3. Which of the following virulence factors contributes to the mucoid phenotype described in the most likely causative agent?

A. Alginate

B. Elastase

C. Exotoxin A

D. Flagella

E. Quorum sensing

4. Which of the following best describes the most common mode of transmission for the causative organism?

A. Air-borne from an infected individual

B. Arthropod-borne from an *Aedes* spp. mosquito

C. Blood-borne from a puncture wound

D. Fecal–oral route

E. Ubiquitous from the environment

5. Which of the following is the best antibiotic treatment strategy for this acute infection?

A. Start oral ciprofloxacin to give the best coverage and the highest compliance

B. Start intravenous colistin due to the high prevalence of resistance in the likely causative organism

C. Start intravenous vancomycin mono-therapy to cover the most likely causative organism

D. Start inhaled tobramycin to treat this contained pulmonary infection

E. Start a combination of intravenous piperacillin–tazobactam and tobramycin to cover the most likely causative organism

Answers and Explanations

1. Correct: *Pseudomonas aeruginosa* (C)

This case describes a young adult with a cough. The patient has a past medical history for a confirmed diagnosis of cystic fibrosis (CF). Sputum culture of a typical CF patient will grow *Staphylococcus aureus* at a young age, replaced by *Pseudomonas aeruginosa* as the patient ages. Other bacteria that may be considered from the sputum of a CF patient include *Haemophilus influenzae*, *Burkholderia cepacia*, and *Stenotrophomonas maltophilia*. Laboratory results indicated growth on blood agar after 24 hours and beta hemolysis, which would be seen for *P. aeruginosa* or *S. aureus* only, of the choices listed (the other organisms listed would require special growth media). The Gram stain image shows gram-negative rods, which is the morphology for *P. aeruginosa*, but not *S. aureus*. Lastly, *P. aeruginosa* are oxidase positive and citrate positive.

A *Legionella pneumophila* cannot be visualized by Gram stain.

B *Mycoplasma pneumoniae* cannot be visualized by Gram stain.

D *S. aureus* are gram-positive cocci, not gram-negative bacilli, as seen in the figure.

E *Streptococcus pneumoniae* are gram-positive cocci, not gram-negative bacilli, as seen in the figure.

2. Correct: Growth with colorless colonies (B)

MacConkey agar is a selective medium that selects for the growth of many gram-negative bacilli (it should be noted that not all gram-negative bacilli will grow on MacConkey agar). This agar contains bile salts that inhibit the growth of gram-positive organisms. MacConkey agar also contains lactose and a pH change indicator. Lactose-fermenting organisms produce acidic by-products, resulting in pink colonies, whereas nonlactose-fermenting organisms can be viewed as colorless colonies. *P. aeruginosa* are gram-negative bacilli, so they will grow on MacConkey agar. However, they are nonlactose-fermenters, so the colonies will be colorless due to the lack of a pH change.

A There are no organisms of medical importance that would have this type of colony morphology on MacConkey agar. Beta-hemolytic bacteria will grow on blood agar with a clearing around the colony indicating hemolysis.

C Lactose-fermenting bacteria, such as *E. coli*, will grow on MacConkey agar as bright pink colonies.

D Gram-positive bacteria, as well as gram-negative bacilli that are not in the Enterobacteriaceae family will not grow on MacConkey agar.

E *Proteus* spp. are bacteria that grow in a typical swarming pattern on many routine media agars.

3. Correct: Alginate (A)

Alginate is the loosely associated capsule that surrounds many clinical isolates of *P. aeruginosa*. It functions to protect the bacteria from phagocytosis, as well as aids in biofilm formation. In the lung environment of CF patients, *P. aeruginosa* produces the polysaccharide alginate that results in a phenotype conversion from nonmucoid to mucoid during chronic colonization.

B Elastase is an enzyme produced by many strains of *P. aeruginosa* that aids in colonization by breaking down host elastin.

C Exotoxin A is an exotoxin that kills host cells through the mechanism of ADP-ribosylating elongation factor 2 (EF-2) and therefore halting protein synthesis, resulting in cell death.

D Most strains of *P. aeruginosa* are motile and produce flagella, but this does not have an effect on the mucoid phenotype.

E *P. aeruginosa* is one of many bacteria that produce quorum sensing molecules, which allows many bacteria to communicate at the population level through the release of chemical signals (autoinducers). Downregulation of quorum sensing may be a result of selective pressure due to the induction of the mucoid phenotype.

4. Correct: Ubiquitous from the environment (E)

P. aeruginosa is found ubiquitously in large quantities in the environment. Most individuals (healthy or otherwise) have evidence of *P. aeruginosa* exposure by the age of 1.

A Air-borne from an infected individual is incorrect. *P. aeruginosa* is not air-borne.

B Arthropod-borne from an *Aedes* spp. mosquito is incorrect. *P. aeruginosa* is not a vector-borne organism.

C Blood-borne from a puncture wound is incorrect. *P. aeruginosa* is not transmitted in the blood.

D Fecal–oral route is incorrect. *P. aeruginosa* is not transmitted via the fecal–oral route.

5. Correct: Start a combination of intravenous piperacillin–tazobactam and tobramycin to cover the most likely causative organism (E)

While there is controversy on the best way to treat acute exacerbations of CF due to *Pseudomonas* infections, the patient described in this case is clearly ill and is in imminent danger due to the infection.

Pseudomonas is the likely causative organism, and resistance is a frequent issue in the treatment of *Pseudomonas* infections; however, this patient has never had a similar infection, and thus while she may have resistance, it is unlikely she has developed resistance to most classes of antipseudomonal antibiotics at this time. A combination of an antipseudomonal beta-lactam (such as piperacillin–tazobactam) and an aminoglycoside (such as tobramycin) is considered appropriate for initial treatment of severe *Pseudomonas* infections.

A Oral ciprofloxacin might be considered for a mild exacerbation, but the use of ciprofloxacin alone for *Pseudomonal* lung infections is generally frowned upon due to the high likelihood of emergence of resistance.

B Colistin is used only in cases where extensive resistance is likely due to its high risk for significant side effects.

C Vancomycin would be appropriate for treatment of methicillin-resistant *S. aureus* (MRSA) but not *Pseudomonas*.

D Given the extent of her illness, this patient is not appropriate for treatment with inhaled antibiotics alone.

Keywords: Cystic fibrosis, *Pseudomonas aeruginosa*, sputum, alginate, mucoid, MacConkey, piperacillin-tazobactam, tobramycin

Case 9

Adult Male with Persistent Cough and Malaise

A 57-year-old otherwise healthy Caucasian male presented to his primary care physician (PCP) in Michigan in mid-February with a fever, cough, and fatigue. He describes that his symptoms have been going on for the past month and indicates that these symptoms have not significantly changed, and he is frustrated that he is not getting better. The PCP asks about sick contacts, and he states that he has been exposed to some children who have had typical winter colds, but they all got better within a week. The PCP asks about travel and other possible exposures and he denies any travel but mentions that he has family all over the world, and he received several gifts from different family members for the holidays. His brother in Florida sent a box of theme park merchandise, his cousin in Arizona sent him a live cactus and some Native American blankets, and his sister in France sent him a few bottles of wine and some jars of French preserves.

Physical examination reveals that the patient's temperature is 38.3°C, blood pressure 110/70 mmHg, and pulse 106 bpm. A chest X-ray is obtained and shows consolidations in the apical regions of the upper right lung. A sputum sample is obtained for laboratory analysis and microscopy with periodic acid–Schiff (PAS) is shown in the figure below.

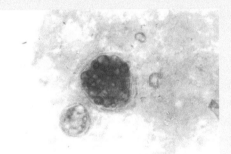

Image courtesy: CDC/ Dr. Gary Carroll

Questions

1. Which of the following organisms is the most likely causative agent?

A. *Aspergillus fumigatus*

B. *Blastomyces dermatitidis*

C. *Coccidioides posadasii*

D. *Histoplasma capsulatum*

E. *Mycobacterium tuberculosis*

2. Which of the following best describes the dimorphic nature of the causative agent?

A. Can synthesize both muscarine and fusariongenin

B. Has a yeast and a mycelial phase

C. Has both septate and aseptate hyphae

D. Infects two different organs at the same time

E. Produces a sporangiophore and mycelium

3. Which of the following diagnostic tests would be the safest to confirm the diagnosis?

A. Culture at 37°C and 25°C

B. Serology with enzyme immunoassay (EIA)

C. Polymerase chain reaction (PCR) of sputum sample

D. Radiography

E. Urine antigen test

4. If examination of medical history of this patient revealed a diagnosis of HIV infection in the past 5 years, which of the following possible complications of infection would be the most cause for worry?

A. Antibiotic-associated colitis

B. Endocarditis

C. Hemolytic uremic syndrome

D. Meningitis

E. Scarlet fever

5. What would be the most appropriate treatment for this patient at this time?

A. Amphotericin B

B. Ceftriaxone

C. Micafungin

D. Fluconazole

E. Symptomatic care only

Answers and Explanations

1. Correct: *Coccidioides posadasii* (C)

The patient's symptoms describe valley fever pneumonia. *Coccidioides posadasii* infections originate from the defined geographical location of Arizona or the southwestern United States (*Coccidioides immitis* is more common in California). The description of the organism as a multinucleate spherule when in a patient sample (at 37°C) also gives a clue as to the fungal pathogen *C. posadasii*. Symptoms of valley fever include cough, fever, fatigue, chest pain, and weight loss. The infection was likely transmitted from either the soil from the cactus plant or dust or sand in the blankets that were received from Arizona, where spores of the organism are commonly found in the desert soil. The patient likely inhaled arthrospores present in the sand, dust, or soil. None of the other choices have the morphology described although some cause similar symptoms.
A *Aspergillus fumigatus* are septate hyphae with dichotomous branching at acute angles.
B *Blastomyces dermatitidis* is a broad-based budding yeast.
D *Histoplasma capsulatum* are small oval brown yeast cells at 37°C.
E *Mycobacterium tuberculosis* are acid-fast bacilli and would not be visualized under nonstained light microscopy.

2. Correct: Has a yeast and a mycelial phase (B)

This patient presents with a *Coccidioides* spp. infection, which are dimorphic fungi. Dimorphic fungi, by definition, have a yeast phase at 37°C and a hyphal or mycelial phase at 25°C.
A, C, D, E None of the other answer choices describe the two phases of a dimorphic fungus. *C. immitis* are dimorphic as multinucleate spherules at 37°C (e.g., at body temperature or when sampled directly from body fluids such as sputum in this case) and septate hyphae with arthrospores at 25°C, or when grown at room temperature.

3. Correct: Serology with enzyme immunoassay (EIA) (B)

Serological testing is routinely done for patients with suspected coccidioidomycosis. Most serologic tests use EIAs for both immunoglobulin M (IgM) and IgG. If EIA is positive, then a confirmatory immunodiffusion test is normally performed, as it gives a qualitative positive for IgG. Other possible tests include immunodiffusion tests (which are less sensitive but more specific), complement fixation tests, or quantitative immunodiffusion tests for IgG.
A While culture will also give a definitive diagnosis, there are safety risks associated because the organism is so easily transmissible and so precautions must be taken. *Coccidioides* spp. are a leading cause of laboratory-acquired infections.
C PCR testing is not routinely available.
D Radiography can be used to confirm a diagnosis of pneumonia but will not give any clues as to the identification of the causative agent.
E A urine antigen test is currently under development, but such a test is not available at this time.

4. Correct: Meningitis (D)

Any individuals with a compromised T-cell immunity are at risk for disseminated *Coccidioides* spp. infection. The most common sites of infection are the central nervous system (CNS), skin, and bone. As such, meningitis is the most common complication of infection among those individuals who are HIV positive.
A Antibiotic-associated colitis is a complication of antibiotic treatment.
B Endocarditis is not a common complication of coccidioidomycosis.
C Hemolytic uremic syndrome is a complication of enterohemorrhagic *Escherichia coli* (EHEC) infections.
E Scarlet fever is a possible complication of a *Streptococcus pyogenes* infection.

5.   Correct: Symptomatic care only (E)

The clinical description is most consistent with acute pulmonary coccidioidomycosis or valley fever. There is nothing in the presentation to suggest severe disease, disseminated disease, acute worsening, or concerning comorbidities. As such for acute valley fever, which usually occurs 1 to 3 weeks after an exposure and can last for months, current recommendations are patient education, observation, and supportive measures only.

A Amphotericin is generally reserved for azole failure or cases with severe immunosuppression.

B Antibiotic treatment such as ceftriaxone would not be appropriate and would not treat *Coccidioides*.

C Micafungin is not used in cases of coccidioidomycosis.

D Antifungal treatment would be appropriate for patients with debilitating disease, evidence of dissemination, frailty due to comorbidities or advanced age, diabetes, or immunosuppression. The generally accepted first-line treatment for nondisseminated severe coccidioidomycosis is fluconazole.

Keywords: Pneumonia, *Coccidioides* spp., fungal, dimorphic, select agent, multinucleate spherule

Case 10

Infant with Severe Congestion

In late January, a mother brought her 5-month-old daughter to her pediatrician because of a fever of 101°F that began the previous night. She reports that the child has had a very runny nose for the last 3 days and has required frequent suction to clear the congestion. The child also has been very sleepy and uninterested in eating or drinking. When asked, the mother reports that the child has had no diarrhea or vomiting but that a dry cough had started earlier that morning.

The child lives with her mother and 3-year-old brother. The mother reports that both children attend daycare three times a week and are watched by their grandmother for 2 other weekdays. Her big brother was diagnosed previously with cough-variant asthma. There are no smokers in the home and no pets. The child is up to date with all recommended vaccinations.

Physical examination identified tachypnea and wheezing; nasal flaring and intercostal retractions were observed on inspiration. Oxygen saturation was low at 91%.

The child was admitted to the hospital and given oxygen. Imaging studies and laboratory tests were ordered including a complete blood count (CBC) with differential that showed a slightly elevated white blood cell (WBC) count with lymphocytosis. A nasopharyngeal swab was collected and sent for respiratory panel testing.

Questions

1. What is the clinical condition that is most likely being experienced by this child?

A. Asthma

B. Bronchiolitis

C. The common cold

D. Influenza

E. Pneumonia

2. Given the patient history, which of the following organisms is most likely the causative agent?

A. *Haemophilus influenzae*

B. Influenza A virus

C. Metapneumovirus

D. Respiratory syncytial virus (RSV)

E. *Streptococcus pneumoniae*

3. How is the causative agent most often spread?

A. Airborne transmission

B. Fomite transmission

C. Foodborne transmission

D. Vector transmission

E. Sexual transmission

4. The F protein of the causative agent is required for infection and is also responsible for which of the following cellular effects?

A. Clumping

B. Granulations

C. Inclusion bodies

D. Syncytia

E. Vacuoles

5. Which of the following is the most appropriate treatment for this patient?

A. Corticosteroids

B. Intravenous immunoglobulin (IVIg)

C. Palivizumab

D. Ribavirin

E. Supportive care

Answers and Explanations

1. Correct: Bronchiolitis (B)

Bronchiolitis is the most common lower respiratory tract infection in infants.

A Asthma is a result of airway edema as compared with bronchiole restriction seen in bronchiolitis. Imaging studies would aid in the differentiation.

C A common cold may have a low-grade fever in children but would not result in breathing difficulty which was observed in the child during the physical examination.

D Influenza infection would result in a much higher fever. Additionally, vomiting and diarrhea may be observed in young children.

E Bronchiolitis can progress to pneumonia, but given the short span of progression, the time of year, and age of the patient, bronchiolitis is the more likely choice.

2. Correct: Respiratory syncytial virus (RSV) (D)

Given the results of the CBC and differential, it is less likely that the infection is bacterial. The PCV13 vaccine for *Streptococcus pneumoniae* is given as a series of three vaccinations at 2, 4, and 6 months. The PCV13 pneumococcal conjugate vaccine covers the same serotypes as the previous PCV7 version with an additional six serotypes. Given the age of the child, the last dose has not yet been issued. The conjugate vaccine for *Haemophilus influenzae* (Hib) is also given in a series of three or four injections beginning at age 2 months then at 4, 6, and 12 to 15 months. Again, only the first two doses would have been received in this case. Both *S. pneumoniae* and *H. influenzae* are a leading cause of pneumonia in unvaccinated children but are not a cause of bronchiolitis. Influenza is a serious disease for children younger than 2 years of age, and yearly vaccination is recommended. However, the vaccine is recommended for those 6 months of age or older. This child would not have received the influenza vaccine. Influenzae A virus does not cause bronchiolitis. Human metapneumovirus (hMPV) is a recently described etiologic agent (2001) for a spectrum of respiratory illnesses including bronchiolitis. Most cases of bronchiolitis (~ 70%) are believed to be caused by RSV, but the contribution of hMPV is now appreciated. Both viruses are negative-stranded RNA viruses belonging to the *Paramyxoviridae* family. While a passive immunization prophylactic treatment using a monoclonal antibody is available for RSV infection, it is generally only offered to infants at high risk of hospitalization due to underlying comorbidities. No vaccine currently is available.

A *H. influenzae* does not cause bronchiolitis.

B Influenzae A virus does not cause bronchiolitis.

C Metapneumovirus can cause bronchiolitis but in this case it is not the causative agent.

E *S. pneumoniae* does not cause bronchiolitis.

3. Correct: Airborne transmission (A)

RSV is highly contagious and is primarily spread by coughing and airborne droplet transmission. Although it is an enveloped virus, it is able to remain viable on contaminated surfaces for several hours.

B Fomite transmission is possible but secondary to airborne transmission.

C, D, E RSV is not transmitted via the foodborne, vector, or sexual transmission routes.

4. Correct: Syncytia (D)

A characteristic cytopathic effect of RSV infection is the formation of syncytia or the fusing of cells to form a single mass with multiple nuclei. The F protein of the virus is essential for fusing the membrane of the virus to endocytic vesicles in cells of the respiratory epithelium after macropinocytosis.

A The F protein of RSV does not cause cell clumping.

B The F protein of RSV does not cause granulations to be formed.

C The F protein of RSV does not cause the formation of inclusion bodies inside of host cells.

E The F protein of RSV does not cause vacuoles to form inside of cells.

5. Correct: Supportive care (E)

In young children (< 2 years of age), supportive care is the treatment of choice for RSV.

A Corticosteroids may be of use in adults and older children, but in randomized trials, they have not been shown to be beneficial in young children.

B A systematic review of studies using IVIg in 2006 failed to show significant benefit.

C Palivizumab is a monoclonal antibody directed against the RSV F protein, but studies have shown no benefit in treatment. It is useful for the prevention of RSV in high-risk children.

D Ribavirin, at one time, was commonly used to treat children with RSV; however, a systematic review of the randomized trials of ribavirin in infants and children did not support its use.

Keywords: Bronchiolitis, respiratory syncytial virus, cytopathic effect, transmission, pneumonia, syncytia

Case 11

Adult Male with Fever, Myalgias, and Respiratory Distress

A 38-year-old otherwise healthy male, is seen in the emergency department in late December with symptoms of 104°F fever, myalgias, and headache for the last 4 days. Currently, he complains of difficulty breathing and lower respiratory pressure. He does not have any upper respiratory congestion but does have a cough. His temperature is 101.5°F after taking 600 mg of ibuprofen and his O_2 saturation on room air is 86%. Crackles and wheezing are heard on auscultation. Laboratory results indicate that the patient has a white blood cell (WBC) count of 7.8×10^9/L (5.8×10^9/L neutrophils; 0.3×10^9/L lymphocytes; 1.7×10^9/L monocytes). An X-ray of his chest is ordered and is normal. A computed tomography (CT) of the chest is done and shows diffuse ground-glass changes. A procalcitonin is sent and the results indicate less than 0.1 ng/mL. When asked, he states that he is not up to date on his yearly vaccinations.

Questions

1. What is the most likely cause of this respiratory infection?

A. Adenovirus

B. Influenza A virus

C. Human metapneumovirus

D. Parainfluenza virus

E. Respiratory syncytial virus

2. Which of the following tests is most commonly used as a first-line test for diagnosing this infection?

A. Antigen detection

B. Bead array–based testing

C. Culture

D. Reverse transcription polymerase chain reaction (RT-PCR)

E. Serology

3. Why is it necessary for this vaccination to be obtained yearly by this patient?

A. The patient has low procalcitonin levels

B. The vaccine requires a booster

C. The virus changes frequently requiring a different vaccine each year

D. The vaccine is therapeutic

E. The patient has an occult immunocompromised state

4. For which of the following is this patient most at risk?

A. Developing a secondary bacterial infection

B. Developing a relapsing viral infection

C. Developing a reaction to additional vaccines

D. Developing an autoimmune nervous system disorder

E. Developing secondary myocarditis

5. Which of the following is the most appropriate treatment for this patient's infection?

A. Amantadine

B. Cidofovir

C. Intravenous immunoglobulin (IVIg)

D. Oseltamivir

E. Ribavirin

Answers and Explanations

1. Correct: Influenza A virus (B)

This is a case of influenza virus infection. Seasonal flu epidemics occur usually from October through May with peaks from December through February, although flu can occur year-round. See figure below for seasonal incidence of viral infections. The human viruses, influenza A and B are responsible for these seasonal outbreaks. Symptoms of acute high fever, severe headache, and body aches are usual along with other common cold symptoms having greater severity. The white blood cell count is also indicative of influenza. Children are more likely to have additional symptoms of vomiting and diarrhea. The severe flu symptoms may last 2 to 5 days, whereas the general cold symptoms of congestion, cough, and fatigue may last 1 to 2 weeks. While any of the viruses listed could in theory be responsible for this infection, given the occurrence is in December, influenza A is the most common of these viruses.

Seasonal Incidence of Viral Infections											
Jan	Feb	Mar	Apr	May	Jun	Jul	Aug	Sep	Oct	Nov	Dec
Adenovirus											
			PIV-3				PIV2, 3				
RSV											
Influenza											
					MPV						

A Adenovirus is less likely because adenovirus rarely presents with myalgia. Infections tend to peak in the fall.

C Human metapneumovirus would rarely be this severe in a patient of this age and health status. The peak season would be later in the year.

D Parainfluenza virus would rarely be this severe in a patient of this age and health status. The peak season would be later in the year.

E Respiratory syncytial virus is less likely because the extremes of age (the young and the elderly) are more likely affected, as well as those individuals with underlying respiratory disease (neither of which are the case for this patient).

2. Correct: Antigen detection (A)

The availability of point-of-care rapid diagnostic tools increases the ease of diagnosis of influenza. There are two types of tests: antigen detection and molecular testing. Antigen detection is more commonly used in outpatient facilities but also frequently used in hospitals. A result turnaround time of 15 to 20 minutes is attainable with the rapid tests as opposed to that of RT-PCR, bead array–based systems, serology, and culture. A caveat to the use of rapid point-of-care testing (POCT) is false-positive and false-negative rates. Depending on the sensitivity of the test, when the prevalence of disease is low, the false-positive rate increases. Conversely, when the prevalence of disease is high, the false-negative rate increases.

B, C, D, E The results of these tests still require consideration of clinical judgment to ascertain a true infection. For these tests, the turnaround time is less rapid than antigen detection and molecular testing. However, results from one of these tests, though slower to obtain, are often required to corroborate the results of the rapid test due to the increased sensitivity of these tests.

3. Correct: The virus changes frequently requiring a different vaccine each year (C)

The influenza vaccine is offered yearly to everyone and is comprised of viral hemagglutinin (H) and neuraminidase (N) antigens. There are commonly three human H antigen types and two neuraminidase types that associate to form multiple viral strain subtypes, e.g., H1N1, while other less common avian strains, for example, H5 or H7, are also capable of infecting humans. The vaccine is typically comprised of antigens for the two strains of seasonal influenza A viruses and one or two strains of influenza B viruses which are predicted to be circulating during influenza season based on what is circulating at the time the vaccines are made. Since there is a several month lead time in the production of the vaccine, sometimes the predictions don't match the reality of what is circulating well and the vaccine is less effective. Vaccines are offered each year as the viruses that circulate change each year. Subtle changes to the epitopes of circulating viruses resulting from acquisition of genetic point mutations can have a major impact on the efficacy of a vaccine. These changes are referred to as antigenic drift and are the main reason the vaccine is given yearly.

A Procalcitonin can be predictive of a bacterial etiology for pneumonia. It is rarely elevated in viral infection. The level has nothing to do with response to vaccines.

B While it is true the immune response generated by the vaccine wanes over time, this is not truly a booster vaccine. With influenza there can also be large-scale genetic changes resulting from the novel reassortment of the H and N antigens referred to as antigenic shift. When an antigenic shift occurs, the vaccines that are generated are ineffective since the changes are so large. This is what led to the 1919 influenza pandemic and the more recent 2009 H1N1 outbreak. When this occurs, rapid development of a new vaccine is needed as was seen in 2009.

D The influenza vaccine is not a therapeutic vaccine, it is preventative.

E This patient is described as otherwise healthy; influenza commonly affects healthy adults; there is no reason to suspect an immunocompromised status in this patient.

4. Correct: Developing a secondary bacterial infection (A)

The primary risk to this patient is post-influenza pneumonia due to bacterial cause. The resolution of the viral infection may reduce the inflammatory response thus setting the stage for subsequent bacterial infection

Keywords: Influenza virus, pneumonia, COPD

progression. The primary pathogens involved are most likely *Staphylococcus aureus, Streptococcus pneumoniae, Streptococcus pyogenes,* and *Haemophilus influenzae.*

B Influenza infections do not "relapse," and so that answer is incorrect.

C This infection is not a reaction to the vaccine, it is a viral infection, so that answer is also incorrect.

D, E Complications of influenza infection do not include autoimmune nervous system disorders or development of a secondary myocarditis.

5. Correct: Oseltamivir (D)

There are three classes of anti-influenza antivirals: amantadines, neuraminidase inhibitors, and a selective inhibitor of influenza community-acquired pneumonia (CAP)-dependent endonuclease. Amantadines inhibit viral uncoating, whereas the neuraminidase inhibitors work by preventing cleavage of the viral particles from the cell. The neuraminidase inhibitors are first-line therapy, and oseltamivir is the most commonly used. Baloxavir is a recently approved inhibitor of influenza CAP-dependent endonuclease. It is not yet considered first line for treatment of influenza, but it could be a reasonable choice in the right person.

A The adamantanes are no longer in use due to near-universal resistance to them by influenza virus.

B Cidofovir has no activity against influenza.

C IVIg might contain protective antibodies against influenza but is not a standard treatment.

E Ribavirin has no activity against influenza.

Case 12 Adult Male with Fever, Chills, and Night Sweats

A 38-year-old male presents to urgent care with fever, chills, malaise, and night sweats. He says he has been feeling weak and has developed a cough. He denies any prior medical problems or sick contacts but mentions he had dental work recently. Examination of the patient's arms is shown in the first figure below. On questioning, he becomes evasive and says he has no idea what they are. The remainder of the physical examination reveals a loud audible heart murmur. The patient is admitted to the hospital, and three blood cultures are taken over a 24-hour period. All three cultures turn positive within less than 12 hours and grow the organism that is shown on the Gram stain (see second figure below). Biochemical testing of the organism reveals that is it both catalase and coagulase positive. An echocardiogram is ordered but not yet performed.

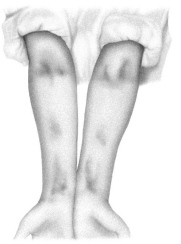

Image courtesy: Lisa D'Angelo

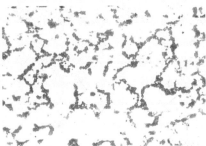

Image courtesy: CDC/ Dr. Richard Facklam

Questions

1. Which of the following organisms is the most likely causative agent?

A. *Enterococcus faecalis*

B. *Staphylococcus aureus*

C. *Staphylococcus epidermidis*

D. *Streptococcus bovis*

E. Viridans group *Streptococcus*

2. Which of the following is the most likely source of infection of the causative agent?

A. Arthropod

B. Endogenous

C. Ingestion

D. Inhalation

E. Needlestick

3. Which of the following valves would be most likely to have a vegetation in this patient when the echocardiogram is performed?

A. Aortic

B. Mitral

C. Pulmonary

D. Tricuspid

4. What is the most appropriate antibiotic to start the patient on initially?

A. Nafcillin

B. Cefazolin

C. Vancomycin

D. Piperacillin–tazobactam

E. Linezolid

5. The patient is started on antibiotics, and when the sensitivities come back for the original antibiotic prescribed, the minimum inhibitory concentration (MIC) is 1, which is considered sensitive. The patient clinically improves over the next 3 days, but despite this, repeat cultures at 48 and 96 hours after initiation of antibiotics are still positive for the same organism and the MIC remains at 1. Which of the following is the most likely cause of the failure to clear the bloodstream infection?

A. Lack of source control

B. Rapid development of resistance to the antibiotic

C. Selection of resistant subpopulations from the initial infection

D. Introduction of a secondary infection

E. Contamination of the blood cultures

Answers and Explanations

1. Correct: *Staphylococcus aureus* (B)

The Gram stain shows gram-positive cocci in clusters, which is a typical microscopic morphology for *Staphylococcus aureus*. Furthermore, *S. aureus* is the only bacteria listed that test catalase and coagulase positive. All of the other organisms listed are possible causative agents for endocarditis, which is the clinical description of this case. *S. aureus* is the most common causative agent of endocarditis (Murdoch et al 2009).

A While *Enterococcus faecalis* are gram-positive cocci, they typically do not have a cluster microscopic arrangement that is shown in the figure. *Enterococcus* spp. are catalase negative.

C While *Staphylococcus epidermidis* are gram-positive cocci, they typically do not have a cluster microscopic arrangement that is shown in the figure. *S. epidermidis* are coagulase negative.

D While *Streptococcus bovis* are gram-positive cocci, they typically do not have a cluster microscopic arrangement that is shown in the figure. *Streptococcus* species are all catalase negative.

E While viridans group *Streptococcus* are gram-positive cocci, they typically do not have a cluster microscopic arrangement that is shown in the figure. *Streptococcus* species are all catalase negative.

2. Correct: Needlestick (E)

In this patient with obvious track marks, *S. aureus* endocarditis is most likely caused by injection drug use. *S. aureus* is the most common pathogen in injection drug users who develop endocarditis.

A Endocarditis is rarely caused by arthropod-borne transmission.

B While the patient notes dental work, the majority of endocarditis after a dental procedure is caused by viridans group of streptococci.

C, D Endocarditis is rarely caused by ingestion or inhalation.

3. Correct: Tricuspid (D)

The tricuspid valve is most commonly affected in an injection drug user with a native value who develops endocarditis.

A, B, C With intravenous (IV) drug use, the mitral is the second most common, the aortic third, and the pulmonic only rarely involved. In most cases of non-IV drug abuse–related endocarditis, the mitral is most common, the aortic the second most common, and the tricuspid infrequent, and the pulmonary valve is very rarely affected during endocarditis.

4. Correct: Vancomycin (C)

This patient has *S. aureus* endocarditis. In IV drug users, it is most commonly methicillin-resistant *S. aureus* (MRSA). Vancomycin is the appropriate choice, is active against MRSA, and first line in the guidelines for empiric treatment of suspected MRSA endocarditis.

A, B are both beta-lactam antibiotics and reasonable choices for methicillin-sensitive *S. aureus* (MSSA) but not for MRSA.

D Piperacillin–tazobactam is also a beta-lactam antibiotic but is primarily used for gram-negative organisms not for *Staphylococcus*.

E Linezolid is active against *S. aureus* and remains active against MRSA but is a bacteriostatic antibiotic against *Staphylococcus* and thus not first line for endocarditis. While there are case reports of using it for endocarditis, it does not have the indication for it.

5. Correct: Lack of source control (A)

The most common reason a patient does not clear a bacteremia associated with endocarditis is lack of source control. This is caused by the inability of the antibiotic to sterilize the vegetation. If the patient is stable and has no other warning signs, sometimes changing the antibiotic or adding a synergistic antibiotic can help clear it. However, in general, failure to sterilize the bloodstream is an indication for surgical intervention and a valve replacement.

B This option is incorrect. Based on the stated MIC in subsequent cultures, there is

no development of resistance seen. Vanco-mycin-resistant *S. aureus* (VRSA) is uncom-mon with less than 20 cases total ever reported, it occurs when the *van A* gene from vancomycin-resistant enterococci (VRE) transfers to MRSA in a patient who is coinfected, which is not described here.
C If a resistant subpopulation were selected out as can be seen in vancomycin-intermediate *S. aureus* (VISA), subsequent cultures should show an elevated MIC as the only thing that would remain in the blood would have an elevated MIC against vancomycin.
D It is unlikely the patient developed a secondary *S. aureus* infection, and if it had an MIC in the sensitive range, it should be cleared as well.
E It is unlikely this is a contaminant; *S. aureus* is rarely a contaminant, and we should not see repeated cultures over mul-tiple days contaminated with the same organism.

Keywords: Endocarditis, heart, *Staphylococcus aureus*, catalase, coagulase, vancomycin, MRSA

Case 13

Child with Bloody Diarrhea

A 5-year-old boy is brought into his pediatrician's office during urgent care hours. His parents state that he developed diarrhea that began as watery and after a couple of days became bloody. He had some cramps but no fever, and his parents were able to keep up on hydration. Initially, they weren't very worried. After about a week, the diarrhea was starting to improve but the patient became lethargic. Physical examination reveals that the patient is afebrile, his heart rate is 110 bpm, his blood pressure is 150/90 mmHg, he is breathing rapidly, and is indeed lethargic. He has slightly pale conjunctiva, slightly icteric sclera, and he withdraws to abdominal palpation.

Upon questioning, the mother mentions that 4 days before the onset of diarrhea, the patient ate at a fast food restaurant with his father and his 12-year-old sister. The father and sister do not appear ill and both ate chicken sandwiches, while the patient ate a cheeseburger at the restaurant. With the exception of that meal, similar meals were consumed by the entire family during the previous several days. Blood is drawn for laboratory work-up. Laboratory results show a hemoglobin of 9 g/dL, a platelet count of 40,000/uL, a total bilirubin of 2.5, and a creatinine level of 2.8 mg/dL. Stool is collected and sent for a battery of cultures, one of which comes back positive after a day.

A Gram stain of the organism from the positive culture is shown in the following figure.

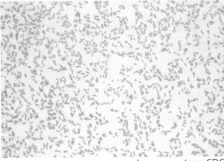

Image courtesy: CDC

Questions

1. Which of the following organisms is the most likely causative agent?

A. *Campylobacter jejuni*

B. *Escherichia coli*

C. Rotavirus

D. *Shigella* spp.

E. *Vibrio cholerae*

2. Which of the following best describes the mechanism of pathogenesis of this agent?

A. Adherence to the colonic mucosa

B. Adherence to the small bowel epithelium

C. Invasion of colonic epithelial cells

D. Production of a cholera-like toxin

E. Production of a Shiga-like toxin

3. Which of the following is the most likely diagnosis accounting for the patient's severe symptoms?

A. Severe dehydration

B. Hemolytic uremic syndrome (HUS)

C. Hemorrhagic colitis

D. Pseudomembranous colitis

E. Typhoid fever

4. The most likely causative agent could be presumptively diagnosed by isolation from the patient's stool and growth on which of the following laboratory media?

A. Hektoen enteric agar (HEA)

B. MacConkey's agar (MAC)

C. Sorbitol MacConkey's agar (SMAC)

D. Thiosulfate citrate bile salts sucrose (TCBS) agar

E. Xylose lysine deoxycholate (XLD) agar

5. What are the most appropriate next steps for the patient at this present time?

A. Send home with instructions to continue with increased oral rehydration therapy

B. Admit the patient to the hospital for observation, hydration, and dialysis as needed

C. Admit the patient to the hospital for treatment with piperacillin–tazobactam and emergent dialysis

D. Admit the patient to the hospital for treatment with intravenous immunoglobulin (IVIg), antitoxin, and plasmapheresis

E. Admit the patient to the hospital for treatment with eculizumab therapy

Answers and Explanations

1. Correct: *Escherichia coli* (B)

Reviewing the patient's characteristics and symptoms will allow identification of the most likely causative agent. Many enteric pathogens can cause dysentery, including *Shigella* spp., *Campylobacter* spp., and *Entamoeba histolytica*. Enterohemorrhagic *E. coli* (EHEC) infections are commonly associated with outbreaks and fast food restaurant ground beef or hamburgers. The mention of a fast food restaurant in this case is a clue to possible *E. coli* O157:H7 and ground beef contamination. EHEC has a 3- to 4-day incubation period (range 1-9 days). Also, the symptoms indicate possible Hemolytic uremic syndrome (HUS), which is a complication of EHEC, thereby making *E. coli* the most likely choice.

A *C. jejuni* is less likely because of the mention of the ground beef and a fast food restaurant. Furthermore, *C. jejuni* are curved gram-negative bacilli while the image shows straight rods. Lastly, *C. jejuni* are not associated with the development of HUS.

C The patient is 5 years of age, so rotavirus is an unlikely causative agent, and the Gram stain indicates a bacterial causative agent.

D There is mention of watery diarrhea, so *Shigella* spp. is likely not the causative agent. *Shigella* spp. infections are more commonly associated with bloody diarrhea.

E The patient does not present with voluminous watery diarrhea, therefore *V. cholerae* is unlikely. Furthermore, the Gram stain shows gram-negative bacilli that do not appear to be comma-shaped, which is characteristic for *V. cholerae*.

2. Correct: Production of a Shiga-like toxin (E)

The causative agent in this case is EHEC, which is also known as Shiga toxin–producing *E. coli* (STEC). EHEC or STEC causes disease via production of a Shiga-like toxin that acts as a cytotoxin to damage the vascular endothelium in the bowel and glomeruli.

A Adherence to the colonic mucosa describes the mechanism of pathogenesis for enteroaggregative *E. coli* (EAggEC or EAEC).

B Adherence to the small bowel epithelium describes the mechanism of pathogenesis for enteropathogenic *E. coli* (EPEC).

C Invasion of colonic epithelial cells is the major mechanism of pathogenesis for enteroinvasive *E. coli* (EIEC).

D Enterotoxigenic *E. coli* (ETEC) produces a cholera-like toxin and colonizes the small bowl during infection.

3. Correct: Hemolytic uremic syndrome (HUS) (B)

This patient is suffering from HUS due to food poisoning caused by EHEC or STEC. Most patients who develop HUS are under the age of 10. HUS is the result of a Shiga-like toxin causing a thrombotic microangiopathy. It is similar to thrombocytopenic purpura but has a significantly better prognosis, especially in young children. HUS occurs in approximately 5% of sporadic *E. coli* O157 infections and can be much more common in certain outbreaks. Acute renal failure occurs in one-half to three-quarters of patients with HUS and 70 to 85% recover with no sequelae. Some patients have lifelong complications including need for dialysis. In 2011, there was an outbreak of colitis linked to *E. coli* O104:H4 due to contaminated sprouted seeds. Nearly 4,000 people were affected with over 50 deaths and 800 cases of HUS. Unusually, the majority of patients in this outbreak were adults.

A Severe dehydration would be seen with low blood pressure, not high as seen in this patient. In addition, this patient is not dehydrated as is stated that his parents were able to keep up with hydration.

C EHEC or STEC may also cause hemorrhagic colitis, but that is not the case for the patient described. The patient described in this case does not show any symptoms consistent with hemmorhagic colitis.

D Pseudomembranous colitis can be seen in *Clostridioides (Clostridium) difficile* infections. This patient's symptoms are not consistent with a *C. difficile* infection.

E Typhoid fever is due to *Salmonella typhi*. This patient does not show any typhoid symptoms.

4. Correct: Sorbitol MacConkey's agar (SMAC) (C)

All of the media listed are used for growth of enteric bacteria. SMAC agar is used routinely to identify *E. coli* O157:H7, as these organisms ferment sorbitol slowly and therefore appear sorbitol negative (non-pigmented) while other *E. coli* species will grow as pink colonies. All sorbitol-negative colonies are then confirmed as *E. coli* using biochemical tests and also tested for a reaction to the O157 antigen. In the case of an outbreak, suspected food contaminants are also tested in a similar way. SMAC is most likely to grow STEC when isolated from stool within the first 6 days following the onset of diarrhea. Other tests that could be used include enzyme-linked immunosorbent assay (ELISA) for Shiga toxin 1 and Shiga toxin 2, and DNA probes for detection of toxin genes.

A HEA is selective and differential for *Salmonella* and *Shigella* species, and would not be useful for identification of *E. coli*.

B MAC is selective and differential for gram-negative enteric bacilli. MAC is not useful to differentiate EHEC or STEC from other enteric pathogens.

D TCBS agar is used for selection of *Vibrio* species and is differential for *V. cholerae* O1.

E XLD agar is a selective growth media used for the isolation of *Salmonella* and *Shigella* species and would not be useful for isolation of EHEC or STEC.

5. Correct: Admit the patient to the hospital for observation, hydration, and dialysis as needed (B)

As HUS disease tends to be self-limited, the most accepted treatment in children is supportive care with dialysis as needed and transfusion in severe anemia. Antibiotics are generally considered to be contraindicated as they may cause additional toxin release and worsening of the HUS.

A HUS is a serious complication of *E. coli* O157 infection and requires admission to the hospital.

C Antibiotics are generally considered to be contraindicated as they may cause additional toxin release and worsening of the HUS.

D IVIg is not used to treat HUS, and there is no specific antitoxin for the Shiga-like toxin. Plasmapheresis is used in adults due to the much more severe outcomes in HUS. It is generally not used in children though there are some data to suggest it may have been used in severe cases.

E Eculizumab is a monoclonal antibody against complement protein C5 and is approved for the treatment of paroxysmal nocturnal hemoglobinuria and atypical HUS. It was used in the 2011 outbreak of *E. coli* O104:H4 in Germany but did not show efficacy nor did it clearly show lack of efficacy either. This was not a true controlled study. Currently, there is no indication for eculizumab therapy in sporadic *E. coli* O157-associated HUS.

Keywords: *Escherichia coli*, EHEC, Enterohemorrhagic, Shiga-like toxin, hemolytic uremic syndrome

Case 14

Child with Stomach Pain and Fever

A 7-year-old boy presents to his pediatrician in June with a 2-day history of fever, abdominal pain, and diarrhea. His parents have kept him home from school due to the symptoms. No one else in the household has diarrhea including his three older brothers and sister. There is no history of unusual foods or exposures and no recent use of antibiotics. He is up to date on his childhood vaccines and there has been no recent travel. The family has three cats, all of which are healthy and have been in the house for at least 5 years. The patient was given a new puppy the week before for his birthday, of which he is very possessive, not letting his brothers or sister play with the puppy and sleeping with the puppy in his bed. The puppy is healthy and was checked by the family vet when they got her. To earn the right to have his puppy, his parents had required him to take care of feeding the cats and cleaning out the litter box for the week before they gave him the puppy.

Physical examination reveals a mildly distressed patient with a diffusely tender abdomen in the left lower quadrant and mild dehydration. His heart rate is 110 bpm, his blood pressure is 100/60 mmHg, and his temperature is 101°F. A stool sample is collected and sent for ova and parasite analysis and culture. Ova and parasite analysis is negative. The stool sample is found to contain fecal leukocytes and trace blood. Cultures on selective media grow an organism that is oxidase positive and grows at 42°C. A Gram stain of the cultured organism is shown in the figure below.

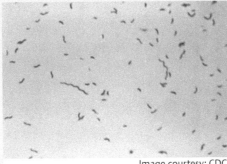

Image courtesy: CDC

Questions

1. Which of the following organisms is the most likely causative agent?

A. *Campylobacter jejuni*

B. *Listeria monocytogenes*

C. *Salmonella enteritidis*

D. *Helicobacter pylori*

E. *Yersinia enterocolitica*

2. For the most likely causative agent, which of the following best describes a symptom of a well-known possible complication of this infection?

A. Ascending attack of peripheral myelin

B. Ulcers in the oral mucosa

C. Rose spots on the abdomen

D. Septic arthritis

E. Vomiting

3. Which of the following bacteriological medias would be required to cultivate the most likely causative agent in the laboratory?

A. CAMPY media

B. MacConkey's agar

C. Tellurite media

D. Mueller–Hinton agar

E. Sorbitol MacConkey's agar

4. Which of the following would have been the most effective action to prevent acquisition of the most likely causative agent in this case?

A. Apply DEET when going outside

B. Wear gloves when emptying the cat litter

C. Wash his hands well after playing with the puppy

D. Avoid eating uncooked shellfish

E. Appropriate vaccination

5. Which of the following is the most appropriate treatment in this case?

A. Admit the patient to the hospital for intravenous (IV) hydration and antibiotics

B. Start oral azithromycin

C. Start antidiarrheal medications

D. Admit the patient to the hospital for plasmapheresis

E. Oral hydration and supportive care only

Answers and Explanations

1. Correct: *Campylobacter jejuni* (A)

Campylobacter spp. are comma-shaped gram-negative rods, as is shown in the figure. They are also oxidase positive and grow best at 42°C in the laboratory.

B *L. monocytogenes* are gram-positive rods, not gram negative as is shown in the figure, and they are oxidase negative.

C *S. enteritidis* are gram-negative rods that are oxidase negative. Transmission of *Salmonella* spp. tends to be associated with contaminated food products and infection outbreaks, which are not mentioned in this case. Furthermore, it would be likely that other family members would also be ill with a *Salmonella* spp. infection.

D *H. pylori* are also oxidase positive and gram-negative curved bacilli, as shown in the figure. *H. pylori* can look very similar to *C. jejuni*, and in fact used to be called *Campylobacter pylori*, but they do not cause a diarrheal illness.

E While *Y. enterocolitica* can also be transmitted by puppies, these organisms are motile at 25°C and nonmotile at 37°C but do not grow well at 42°C.

2. Correct: Ascending attack of peripheral myelin (A)

This patient has an infection with *C. jejuni*, which causes bloody diarrhea and has been linked to Guillain–Barré syndrome and reactive arthritis. Guillain–Barré syndrome is a cause of acute peripheral neuropathy that causes progressive weakness. Most patients have a preceding viral or gastrointestinal (GI) illness. Cytomegalovirus (CMV) has also been associated with this syndrome.

B Ulcers in the oral mucosa are a symptom of hand-foot-and-mouth disease which is most commonly caused by Coxsackie A virus, not *Campylobacter* infections.

C Rose spots are often seen with typhoid fever (caused by *Salmonella typhi*), which also causes bloody diarrhea and is gram-negative. However, it is hydrogen sulfide positive, does not ferment lactose, and is oxidase negative.

D Septic arthritis is a complication of *Neisseria gonorrhoeae,* which does not cause GI symptoms, and is sexually transmitted.

E *Campylobacter* spp. infections do not normally involve vomiting. Food poisoning caused by *Staphylococcus aureus* and some strains of *Bacillus cereus* can be associated with vomiting.

3. Correct: CAMPY media (A)

Campylobacter spp. require specialized media for growth in the laboratory at 42°C in microaerophilic conditions. The media used to cultivate *Campylobacter* spp. is CAMPY media.

B MacConkey's agar is selective and differential media for many enteric bacteria that are not fastidious. *Campylobacter* spp. do not grow on MacConkey's agar.

C Tellurite media is a selective media for growth of *Corynebacterium diphtheriae*.

D *H. pylori* can grow on Mueller–Hinton agar when supplement with 10% blood.

E Sorbitol MacConkey's agar is used to identify enterohemorrhagic *Escherichia coli* (EHEC). Blood agar is used for routine culture of nonfastidious bacteria, but *Campylobacter* spp. do not grow on this media.

4. Correct: Wash his hands well after playing with the puppy (C)

While the most common source of *C. jejuni* in humans is transmission from undercooked poultry which is almost universally contaminated with *C. jejuni*, it would be unusual for a young child to be the only one in a household who develops the infection from such an exposure. *C. jejuni* can be transmitted from puppies that act as carriers for these bacteria even when not sick from it themselves. In this case, the patient had a brand new puppy that was his and he was possessive of it, not letting the others play with it.

A The infection cannot be transmitted by arthropods, so the application of DEET would have no effect on transmission as it would for arthropod-borne infections.

B Cats are not a known carrier of *Campylobacter* spp.

D Contaminated seafood is also not a common transmission vehicle for these bacteria.

E There is no vaccine available for prevention of *Campylobacter* spp. infections. Other prevention methods include avoiding undercooked poultry and unpasteurized dairy products. Utensils, cutting boards, and other food preparation tools for raw poultry should be cleaned thoroughly.

5. Correct: Oral hydration and supportive care only (E)

Most cases of *Campylobacter* spp. in humans are self-limited and only last a few days. In general, even in young children, no specific treatment other than to make sure they drink enough to not become dehydrated is needed.

A The patient does not have any signs of severe dehydration which would lead to the need to hospitalize him and give IV fluids.

B Azithromycin can be used as a treatment in more severe cases and can shorten the illness.

C Antidiarrheal medications are not typically recommended and can actually worsen the illness.

D Plasmapheresis would be used not to treat *C. jejuni* but might be used to treat Guillain–Barré syndrome if it develops.

Keywords: *Campylobacter jejuni*, Gullain-Barré syndrome, oxidase positive, comma-shaped, diarrhea, abdominal pain

Case 15

Outbreak of Diarrheal Illness

One hundred and twenty-eight passengers of a full 2,000-passenger capacity cruise ship (6.4% of the passengers) develop abrupt-onset vomiting, upset stomach, and profuse watery diarrhea. An additional 43 passengers (2.2% of passengers) complain of a slight fever and mild watery diarrhea. Stool samples are collected from 10 of the patients and neither blood nor mucous is observed. Fecal leukocytes are not seen. Stool cultures from the 10 patients did not grow any consistent pathogens on routine media. Most of the passengers recover in 2 to 3 days, but each day for the next 5 days new passengers fall ill until nearly 20% of the passengers and 5% of the crew were affected. Two children under the age of 1 year required hospitalization due to severe dehydration.

Questions

1. Which of the following organisms is the most likely the causative agent of this outbreak?

A. Calicivirus

B. *Campylobacter jejuni*

C. Cytomegalovirus (CMV)

D. Enterotoxigenic *Escherichia coli* (ETEC)

E. *Salmonella typhi*

2. Which of the following describes the genome of the most likely causative agent of this outbreak?

A. Circular double-stranded DNA

B. Double-stranded RNA

C. Linear double-stranded DNA

D. Negative-sense single-stranded RNA

E. Positive-sense single-stranded RNA

3. If the source of the infection could be identified, which of the following would be the most likely source of infection for the outbreak?

A. Cream-filled desserts

B. Fresh fruit

C. Poultry

D. Unpasteurized milk

E. Water

4. An epidemiological investigation is initiated and strain typing is performed to further identify and control the causative pathogen of the outbreak. Which of the following methods would most likely be used for diagnosis and identification of the causative strain?

A. Culture on MacConkey's agar

B. Electron microscopy

C. Gram stain and dark-field microscopy

D. Reverse transcriptase polymerase chain reaction (RT-PCR)

E. Serology, including convalescent titers

5. In addition to keeping up the hydration of the affected passengers, what is the most important policy the cruise ship can implement?

A. Isolate all affected passengers and crew to their rooms

B. Require all passengers and crew to use Pepto-Bismol with each meal

C. Disembark all passengers and clean the ship with bleach

D. Do not let any new passengers onboard at any port

E. Encourage frequent hand hygiene among the passengers and strict hand hygiene among food service staff

1. Correct: Calicivirus (A)

Caliciviruses are the most common outbreak cause of nonbacterial gastroenteritis worldwide. They can cause epidemics in all age groups, but the young and the old are more likely to experience more severe symptoms and complications. Human caliciviruses include norovirus (previously referred to as Norwalk virus) and sapovirus. This question describes a foodborne illness outbreak in a closed environment where individuals are living in close quarters. The lack of blood and fecal leukocytes suggests a noninflammatory gastroenteritis, thereby limiting the correct choices to calicivirus and ETEC.

B *Campylobacter jejuni* cause inflammatory gastro-enteritis.

C CMV does not cause outbreaks.

D Calicivirus infections are more commonly associated with outbreaks in closed environments, such as cruise ships. Furthermore, over half of the cases involved vomiting, which is also more common for calicivirus infection. Therefore, calicivirus is a more likely answer than ETEC.

E *Salmonella typhi* also cause inflammatory gastro-enteritis.

2. Correct: Positive-sense single-stranded RNA (E)

Norovirus is a virus that has a positive-sense, single-stranded RNA genome (+ssRNA). The genome can act directly as a messenger RNA (mRNA) as well as the genome during the viral life cycle.

A Bacterial genomes are circular double-stranded DNA (dsDNA).

B Some viral genomes such as rotavirus are double-stranded RNA (dsRNA).

C Some bacterial (*Borrelia* spp.) and viral genomes such as poxviruses, have some linear double-stranded DNA (dsDNA).

D The flu and RSV virus genomes are negative-sense single stranded RNA (-ssRNA).

3. Correct: Fresh fruit (B)

Most norovirus infections are spread person-to-person, especially on cruise ships. Unwashed fresh fruits or vegetables and/or shellfish contaminated at the source are the most commonly implicated foods of norovirus outbreaks, when a source can be determined.

A Cream-filled desserts are more commonly implicated in *Bacillus cereus* or *Staphylococcus aureus* food poisoning.

C Undercooked poultry is more often associated with *Salmonella* infections.

D *Listeria monocytogenes* is often associated with illness due to unpasteurized milk.

E Norovirus is not generally transmitted via water.

4. Correct: Reverse transcriptase polymerase chain reaction (RT-PCR) (D)

As for most viral infections, nucleic acid-based detection methods are commonly used for identification, along with clinical signs and symptoms and negative results for other tests (in this case, such as rotavirus). In addition, techniques such as RT-PCR can detect a low stool viral load of less than 100 particles/g, making it a good test to use for outbreak situations. Nucleic acid tests have the added advantages of being able to provide genomic information such as strain typing, and can be used with food and environmental samples to identify the source of contamination.

A Viruses do not grow on MacConkey's plates, only some gram-negative bacteria grow on these plates.

B While viruses can be visualized by electron microscopy, strains cannot be distinguished by microscopy methods.

C Viruses cannot be visualized by Gram stain or dark-field microscopy. Only bacteria and fungi can be visualized using those methods.

E Serology can be useful for determining infection of individuals but is not often used for epidemiological studies.

5. Correct: Encourage frequent hand hygiene among the passengers and strict hand hygiene among food service staff (E)

The spread of norovirus is person to person via the fecal-oral route. The most common ways this occurs is eating food or drinking liquids contaminated with norovirus, touching contaminated surfaces and then putting unwashed fingers in the mouth, and sharing food or utensils with an affected individual. All of these are best handled with improved hand hygiene. Prevention of person-to-person spread is best achieved by restricting access to contaminated surfaces.

A It is not reasonable to isolate all affected passengers and crew to their rooms, plus this does not address the asymptomatic individuals.

B Pepto-Bismol does not have an effect on this viral infection.

C, D These measures will remove the virus from surfaces but not the people.

Keywords: Diarrhea, foodborne, norovirus, RNA virus

Case 16

Hospitalized Adult Female Who Develops Diarrhea

A 29-year-old female is hospitalized for community-acquired pneumonia (CAP) and treated with 7 days of ceftriaxone and azithromycin. While hospitalized, she improves on these antibiotics and she started breathing better over the next 3 days, resolves her chest pain and fever, and her white blood cell count, which was 15,000 cells/μL on admission, returns to normal at 6,700 cells/μL. However, on the fifth day of hospitalization, she develops a severe watery diarrhea where she is going to the bathroom 20 times per day. It is associated with crampy bilateral lower quadrant pain. She has a temperature of 102.4°F and routine laboratories reveal a white blood cell count of 23,500 cells/μL. A stool test is done that establishes the diagnosis.

Questions

1. Which of the following organisms is the most likely causative agent?

A. *Campylobacter jejuni*
B. *Clostridioides difficile*
C. *Helicobacter pylori*
D. *Salmonella typhi*
E. *Yersinia enterocolitica*

2. Which of the following would be the most likely test to establish the cause of this woman's diarrhea?

A. Polymerase chain reaction (PCR) for toxins
B. Gram stain and culture
C. Urease breath test
D. Fecal lactoferrin
E. Quantitative bacterial cultures

3. Which of the following biological features allow for the spread of this organism from the environment?

A. An envelope
B. A thick capsule
C. A nonenveloped capsid
D. A spore
E. Toxin production

4. Which of the following describes the major mode of pathogenesis of the infection described for this patient?

A. Endotoxin production
B. Exotoxin production
C. Induction of host cyclic adenosine monophosphate (cAMP)
D. Invasion of the gastric mucosa
E. Urease production

5. The patient is treated for her diarrhea for 14 days and it resolves. She is discharged from the hospital and is doing well but 3 weeks later develops profound watery diarrhea again and becomes dehydrated leading to her readmission to the hospital. The most likely reason she developed this second episode of diarrhea is due to which of the following events?

A. Unrelated to the original infections
B. A delayed necrosis of the colon due to toxins
C. Inappropriate duration of the initial treatment
D. She has been reinfected with the original pathogen
E. Surviving spores have re-established the infection

Answers and Explanations

1. Correct: *Clostridioides difficile* (B)

The clinical scenario described is typical of a *C. difficile* infection (*Clostridioides difficile* is formerly known as *Clostridium difficile*), otherwise known as antibiotic-associated pseudomembranous colitis. A Gram stain is shown in the following figure.

The patient is hospitalized and taking broad-spectrum antibiotics. Antibiotic use is the major risk factor for *C. difficile* infections. The antibiotic treatment affects the normal flora of the gastrointestinal tract, thereby making an environment more hospitable to overgrowth by *C. difficile*. Furthermore, these bacteria are often hospital-acquired and are able to withstand harsh conditions such as hospital cleaning supplies due to the ability to form spores. All of the other options are often community-acquired rather than hospital-acquired. Lastly, the Gram stain shows gram-positive rods, which is the morphology of *C. difficile* but not any of the other answer choices listed.

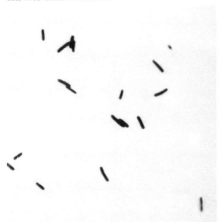

Image courtesy: CDC/Dr. Holdeman

A *Campylobacter jejuni* is often associated with transmission from puppies and gastrointestinal symptoms.
C *Helicobacter pylori* is associated with gastrointestinal ulcers.
D *Salmonella typhi* transmission is usually food-associated, and symptoms are often systemic.

E *Yersinia enterocolitica* often presents similar to appendicitis, and transmission is usually food-associated.

2. Correct: Polymerase chain reaction (PCR) for toxins (A)

The case describes a *C. difficile* infection. Because it is often difficult to isolate the organism directly, diagnosis of *C. difficile* is routinely done by PCR for the toxin genes A and B.
B This option is incorrect because Gram stain and culture often cannot be successfully achieved due to the fact that *C. difficile* is an anaerobe, and the gastrointestinal tract contains so many other normal flora organisms. Gram stain and culture are nearly always inconclusive due to the large number of organisms present.
C The urease breath test is used to diagnose *H. pylori*, not *C. difficile* infections.
D Fecal lactoferrin is a marker of intestinal inflammation, but is not specific for *C. difficile* infections.
E Quantitative bacterial cultures do not identify the causative agent, the test would only be informative of the number of organisms present.

3. Correct: A spore (D)

C. difficile is an aerobic gram-positive rod. It is able to produce spores when in harsh environments, such as heat, acid, and antibiotics, in order to survive. Transmission is often in the hospital setting because the spores are able to survive treatment by most common hospital cleaning products that kill most other bacterial pathogens. *C. difficile* is highly transmissible via the fecal–oral route by ingestion of spores and the bacteria can be found on personal items in patient rooms, clothing, hands, and stethoscopes of health care workers.
A The ability to form an envelope is common to all bacteria and many viruses but does not specifically allow for survival in the hospital environment. Lipopolysaccharide (LPS) is a common component of gram-negative cell walls, and is not a component of a *C. difficile* cell wall.
B The ability to produce a capsule allows many encapsulated bacteria to avoid

phagocytosis. *C. difficile* do not typically produce capsules.

C A nonenveloped capsid allows many viruses to survive harsh environments, but *C. difficile* is a bacterium, not a virus.

E While *C. difficile* are able to produce toxins, this ability does not enable the bacteria to survive in the environment.

4. Correct: Exotoxin production (B)

C. difficile infections are primarily toxin-mediated diseases. The organisms produce small quantities of toxin A and toxin B, which are exotoxins. Only when the numbers of organisms that colonize the gastrointestinal tract reach high numbers, the effects of these exotoxins result in cytotoxic effects on human cells.

A *C. difficile* are gram-positive, and so they do not produce endotoxin (LPS), so A is incorrect.

C Toxins A and B do not act by induction of host cAMP, so option C is incorrect. Toxin A is an enterotoxin that alters host cell permeability through the MAP-kinase pathway. Toxin B is a cytotoxin that results in host cell death via the small GTPase Rho proteins.

D *C. difficile* does not invade the gastric mucosa. Many gastrointestinal pathogens, such as *S. typhi*, *Shigella* spp., enterohemorrhagic *Escherichia coli* (EHEC), and *C. jejuni* are able to invade the gastric mucosa.

E *C. difficile* does not produce the enzyme urease. *H. pylori* produces urease during infection.

5. Correct: Surviving spores have re-established the infection (E)

C. difficile is a spore-forming organism, and even with appropriate treatment, there is an approximately 25% chance of relapse. This relapse occurs when surviving spores, which are unaffected by antibiotic treatment, germinate and reestablish the infection before the normal beneficial bacteria can reestablish in the colon which would keep the *C. difficile* infection under control. Many patients who relapse also have a decreased ability to form antibodies against *C. difficile*, and a recently approved adjuvant therapy for preventing the relapse of *C. difficile* infection is a monoclonal antibody against *C. difficile* toxin B.

A While it is certainly possible that a patient with recent *C. difficile* infection can develop a different infection or cause of acute diarrhea, there is nothing given in the question that points toward that, and the timing is appropriate for a relapse of the original *C. difficile* infection.

B This option is incorrect, as a delayed necrosis of the colon from the toxins is not a feature of the pathogenesis of *C. difficile*. Some patients will develop a lesser diarrhea following an episode of *C. difficile* infection, but this is due to a postinfectious irritable bowel and is not consistent with the profound watery diarrhea described in the question.

C This is incorrect, the appropriate duration of treatment for *C. difficile* is 10 to 21 days.

D This option is incorrect. While patients can be reinfected with *C. difficile* at a later date, relapse is much more likely given the time frame described in the question.

Keywords: *Clostridioides (Clostridium) difficile*, pseudomembranous colitis, antibiotics, gastrointestinal, hospitalized, nosocomial, toxin

Case 17 HIV-Positive Male with Diarrhea

A 32-year-old male was seen by his primary care physician with symptoms of severe stomach cramps, foul-smelling watery diarrhea, and headache that began 8 days earlier. His past medical history indicates a positive diagnosis of HIV. His current HIV therapy is emtricitabine, efavirenz, and tenofovir. His last HIV viral load 2 months ago was undetectable. His CD4 count at that time was 536 cells/mm³. He reports no recent travel or exposure to small children. He did mention that his partner, who is HIV negative, had traveled to Southeast Asia recently on business but doesn't report any symptoms. A microscopic evaluation revealed the organism that is shown in the following figure.

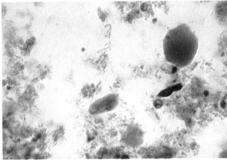

Image courtesy: CDC

Questions

1. Which of the following organisms is most likely the cause of these symptoms?

A. *Campylobacter jejuni*

B. Cytomegalovirus

C. *Giardia lamblia*

D. Norovirus

E. *Salmonella typhi*

2. Which of the following tests is the gold standard for confirming infection with this organism?

A. Culture and stain

B. Fecal immunoassay

C. Ova and parasite (O&P) examination

D. Polymerase chain reaction (PCR)

E. Rapid immunochromatographic assay

3. Which of the following stages of this organism is found almost exclusively in the human intestine?

A. Cyst

B. Gametocyte

C. Merozoite

D. Spore

E. Trophozoite

4. By which structure does this organism adhere to the intestinal wall?

A. Axoneme

B. Flagella

C. Marginal plate

D. Parabasal body

E. Ventral disk

5. Which of the following is the most appropriate treatment for the patient at this time?

A. Bismuth

B. Ciprofloxacin

C. Ganciclovir

D. Imodium

E. Metronidazole

Answers and Explanations

1. Correct: *Giardia lamblia* (C)

Infection by all of the organisms listed can result in intestinal infection in humans. Described in this case is an infection with the parasite *Giardia lamblia*. *Giardia* spp. are transmitted via the fecal–oral route. Giardiasis results in watery diarrhea, abdominal cramps, bloating, and nausea. While *Giardia* spp. infections do occur in the United States, prevalence rates in developing countries are much higher. Those at greatest risk of infection are children, close household contacts, those exposed to contaminated water sources, and men who have sex with men. The majority of adult infections are asymptomatic. For those who become symptomatic, symptoms appear 1 to 3 weeks after infection. There is a strong correlation of giardiasis with HIV infection.
A No gram-negative bacilli are visualized, eliminating the bacterial options, including the gram-negative curved bacilli, *Campylobacter jejuni*. In addition, the foul smell is not characteristic of infections by *C. jejuni*.
B The figure shows the causative organism, which eliminates a viral causative agent. Therefore cytomegalovirus is incorrect. In addition, the foul smell is not characteristic of infections by CMV.
D The figure shows the causative organism, which eliminates a viral causative agent. Therefore norovirus is incorrect. In addition, the foul smell is not characteristic of infections by notovirus.
E No gram-negative bacilli are visualized, eliminating the bacterial options, including the gram-negative bacilli, *Salmonella typhi*. In addition, *S. typhi* infections are rarely associated with foul smelling diarrhea.

2. Correct: Ova and parasite (O&P) examination (C)

The O&P is considered the gold standard for *Giardia* diagnosis. The test consists of microscopic examination of slide preparations from three stool specimens collected from the patient at 2- to 3-day intervals.

The reason for multiple samples being required is because the organism is shed irregularly and may be missed with only one specimen evaluation.
A Microscopic analysis can detect additional organisms that may be contributing to the disease. However *Giardia* is not routinely cultured.
B While antigen immunoassays are shown to have similar sensitivity to microscopic detection, antigen tests may not detect all forms of the parasite.
D PCR is useful for subtype identification.
E Rapid immunoassays are replacing microscopy as the routine diagnostic method and may replace O&P as the gold standard in the future. Microscopy requires expert evaluation, whereas the rapid tests are generally easier to execute.

3. Correct: Trophozoite (E)

The trophozoite form of the organism is found primarily in the human intestine. The trophozoite has a characteristic pear shape with two nuclei and central karyosomes that give the organism a face-like appearance observed in microscopy (as shown in the figure).
A The cyst form is most often detected in feces.
B Gametocytes are more commonly associated with *Plasmodium* spp, the causative agent of malaria.
C Merozoites are more commonly associated with *Plasmodium* spp, the causative agent of malaria.
D Spores are produced by many human pathogens but are not normally found in the human intestine.

4. Correct: Ventral disk (E)

Giardia spp. attach to the epithelium of the small intestine using its ventral disk. This appendage acts like a suction device and is a rigid structure that occupies approximately two-thirds of the ventral surface of the organism.
A, B, C, D Other structures listed are not used by *Giardia* spp. for attachment or are not structures associated with this parasite.

5. Correct: Metronidazole (E)

The most common, effective treatments for *Giardia* spp. infections include metronidazole, tinidazole, and nitazoxanide, with metronidazole being the most commonly used therapy. There are other alternatives but not all are available commonly in the United States and most have not been well studied.

A Ciprofloxacin doesn't treat *Giardia* infections.
B Bismuth doesn't treat *Giardia* infections.
C Ganciclovir is an antiviral agent.
D Imodium just treats diarrhea but is not specific for *Giardia*.

Keywords: Parasite, diarrhea, HIV, STD, metronidazole, giardiasis

Case 18

Adult with Jaundice

A 63-year-old male sees his primary care physician for symptoms of fatigue, arthralgia, some nausea, and swelling in his legs. On physical examination, his vital signs are normal. Some yellowing of the skin and eyes is noted. Hepatomegaly is noted on palpitation. Total bilirubin level is determined to be 2.6 mg/dL. Aminotransferase values were three times the upper limit of normal. He is currently on hydrochlorothiazide for hypertension. He has been married for 41 years to his high school sweetheart. He reports no travel outside of the United States. He drinks alcohol rarely and has no history of drug use. He has had no prior hospitalizations and no body piercings. He does have a large tattoo on his left bicep that he received when he was 28 years of age.

Questions

1. Which virus is most likely the cause of this patient's symptoms?

A. Cytomegalovirus (CMV)

B. Hepatitis A virus (HAV)

C. Hepatitis B virus (HBV)

D. Hepatitis C virus (HCV)

E. Hepatitis D virus (HDV)

2. Which of the following tests would be used to detect a current viral infection?

A. Antibody test

B. Clinical evaluation

C. Cytotoxicity assay

D. Nucleic acid test

E. Rapid point-of-care test

3. Which of the following conditions is of most immediate concern for a chronically infected individual?

A. Cirrhosis

B. Dementia

C. Death

D. Immunodeficiency

E. Liver cancer

4. Which of the following is the cellular location of viral replication for this virus?

A. Clathrin-coated pits

B. Endoplasmic reticulum

C. Membranous web

D. Nucleus

E. Plasma membrane

5. Which of the following additional tests are needed to aid in initial treatment choice?

A. Anti-ribavirin antibody level

B. Gamma-glutamyltransferase

C. Interferon level and subtype

D. Quantitative viral antibody level

E. Viral genotype

Answers and Explanations

1. Correct: Hepatitis C virus (HCV) (D)

This is a case of chronic hepatitis C viral infection. Risk factors for HCV are primarily blood-to-blood transmission and infection by contaminated needles. A history of tattooing prior to the 1990s increases the risk of infection as the virus was unknown at that time. There still continues to be an elevated risk of virus acquisition from tattooing especially for tattoos acquired from private artists as opposed to commercial salons. In general, the risk of chronic HCV is greatest for individuals from the baby boomer generation. This is thought to be due to the high prevalence of the virus, lack of knowledge of the virus, and contamination of the blood supply during the 1960s through the 1980s.

A CMV does not cause chronic hepatitis.

B Hepatitis A virus is food-borne.

C Hepatitis B viruses are most commonly transmitted through contaminated needles of intravenous (IV) drug users or other blood transmission and are not highly associated with the practices of tattoo artistry.

E Hepatitis D viruses are associated with Hepatitis B infections. In fact, HDV can only cause infection via a co-infection or super-infection with HBV.

2. Correct: Nucleic acid test (D)

An acute HCV infection results in detectable viral nucleic acid but may not yet have detectable antibody to the virus (recall that antibody production follows exposure of the immune system to foreign antigen). A chronic infection (such as is described in this case) would have both detectable antibody and nucleic acid in most scenarios. Someone who was once infected and cleared the virus will be antibody positive and nucleic acid negative. Therefore, a current infection (such as the chronic infection described here) requires detection of viral nucleic acid in order to distinguish from the other scenarios.

A An acute HCV infection results in detectable viral nucleic acid but may not yet have detectable antibody to the virus (recall that antibody production follows exposure of the immune system to foreign antigen). A chronic infection (such as is described in this case) would have both detectable antibody and nucleic acid in most scenarios. Someone who was once infected and cleared the virus will be antibody positive and therefore an antibody test would not be suitable for diagnosis.

B Clinical evaluation is useful to identify hepatitis but is not sensitive enough to distinguish HBV from other hepatitis infections.

C A cytotoxicity assay is not routinely utilized to identify HBV infection.

E At present, there aren't any FDA-approved rapid point-of-care tests for HCV.

3. Correct: Cirrhosis (A)

Approximately 75 to 85% of HCV-infected individuals will become chronically infected. Of those individuals with a chronic HCV infection, 10 to 15% will progress to cirrhosis. Additionally, 5 to 30% of those with cirrhosis will experience liver decompensation by 10 years following the diagnosis of cirrhosis.

B While HCV has been associated with neurocognitive disorders, primary dementia is not one of them.

C While the mortality rate in the extreme case does increase significantly, the immediate concern of chronic infection is liver cirrhosis.

D HCV itself does not cause immunodeficiency.

E Hepatocellular carcinoma (HCC) is also a significant risk for a chronically HCV-infected patient. HCC generally occurs only after 20 years or more of HCV infection and after development of cirrhosis or advanced fibrosis. HCC is nearly 20 times more prevalent in HCV-infected cirrhotics than it is in HCV-negative individuals.

4. Answers: Membranous web (C)

HCV is a positive-sense single-stranded Hepacivirus of the family *Flaviviridae*. Replication of this virus occurs in the cytoplasm of infected hepatocytes. Viral proteins reorganize the host cell membranes to construct a membranous region called the membranous web. This web creates a compartmentalized area whereby viral replication can occur, perhaps protected from detection by the cellular pattern recognition receptors.

A Hepatitis B virus does not replicate in clathrin-coated pits.

B HBV does not replicate in the endoplasmic reticulum.

D HBV does not replicate in the nucleus. Herpesviruses replicate in the nucleus.

E HBV does not replicate in the plasma membrane.

5. Correct: Viral genotype (E)

The treatment of HCV has previously been complex and difficult with high failure rates and treatments with high levels of significant side effects. Prior regimens were centered around interferon as an immunomodulatory agent. Since the advent of direct-acting antiviral agents, treatments now have over 90% plus success rate with shorter treatment courses and greatly reduced side effects. There are numerous tests needed before initiating treatment, but the first test needed to help guide the treatment choice is to determine the genotype of the HCV. HCV has six genotypes, and different regimens are indicated for each subtype in order to achieve optimal treatment outcomes.

A, B, C, D These options are incorrect because the only one of these tests that impacts the choice of treatment is genotype.

Keywords: Hepatitis, jaundice, RNA virus, HCV

Case 19

Adult with Right Upper Quadrant Pain

A 58-year-old Asian-American male who has been undergoing systemic chemotherapy for lymphoma for the past several months comes to his family physician with concerns of pain in the right upper quadrant of his abdomen. The patient also describes nausea and occasional vomiting. He is currently off cycle for his cancer treatment. He also reports increased fatigue for the last 2 weeks. Physical examination was remarkable for hepatomegaly. A metabolic panel was ordered that identified alanine aminotransferase levels approximately five times above the upper limit of normal. Blood testing also identified low platelets and prolonged prothrombin time. Transient elastography measurements identified liver stiffness within the normal range. A hepatitis viral serology panel is performed and results are shown in **Table 19.1.**

Table 19.1 Results of hepatitis viral serology panel

Serological Marker	Result
HAV IgM	Negative
HAV IgG	Negative
Anti-HBs	Negative
HBc IgM	Negative
HBc IgG	Positive
HBsAg	Positive
HBeAg	Positive
HBV DNA	7.5×10^8 copies/mL
HCV IgM	Negative
HCV IgG	Negative
HEV IgM	Negative
HEV IgG	Negative

Questions

1. Which of the following is most likely the current stage of this patient's disease?

A. Acute infection, early phase

B. Acute infection, recovery phase

C. Chronic infection

D. Cleared infection

E. Vaccinated individual

2. Given this patient's infection and current condition, for which of the following is the patient most at risk of developing?

A. Atherosclerosis

B. Cirrhosis

C. Hepatic cancer

D. Fulminant renal failure

E. Fulminant liver failure

3. What strategy would have been most effective in preventing the infection from flaring in this patient after he received chemotherapy?

A. Avoidance of all alcohol for the duration of treatment

B. Prophylaxis with anti-HBV immunoglobulin

C. Prophylaxis with lamivudine

D. Vaccination against hepatitis B virus (HBV)

E. There is no proven preventative strategy

4. Which of the following viral enzymes is a therapeutic target?

A. Helicase

B. Integrase

C. Protease

D. Reverse transcriptase

E. Thymidine kinase

5. Which of the following is the most appropriate treatment for this patient at this time?

A. Anti-HBV immunoglobulin

B. Lamivudine

C. Ledipasvir/sofosbuvir

D. Liver transplant

E. Tenofovir

Answers and Explanations

1. Correct: Chronic infection (C)

This is an infection caused by HBV, a *Hepadnaviridae* virus. Reactivation of HBV is well documented in the context of cancer chemotherapy. Individuals with chronic HBV infection as well as those who have cleared a previous infection according to diagnostic markers have a risk for reactivation. Alanine aminotransferase levels as an indication of liver function can become elevated weeks after receiving chemotherapy and preceded by viral reactivation and increase in viral load. The risk of reactivation of HBV varies depending on the type of infection the patient had prior to receiving chemotherapy. Reactivation can occur in both hepatitis B virus surface antigen (HBsAg)-positive and negative patients. Hepatitis C virus (HCV) can also be reactivated in the context of chemotherapy. HCV is a Hepacivirus of the *Flaviviridae* family and is much more common than HBV in the United States; however, the serology for HCV is negative for the patient in this case. Additionally, HCV is less common in the Asian American population with 0.08 cases per 100,000 population as compared with the white population having 0.77 cases. Hepatitis A virus (HAV) is a Hepatovirus of the *Picornaviridae* family. Although it may cause similar symptoms, HAV results in a self-limited acute infection that resolves, and the serology is negative in this case. It is usually transmitted by contaminated food sources and has no specific relationship to cancer chemotherapy. Hepatitis E virus is of the family *Hepeviridae* and is transmitted by the fecal–oral route. The serology for this virus is also negative.

Serological testing for HBV is useful to determine timing of presentation. Individuals who are HBs and HBe antigen positive are in an active infection stage, and if they have HB core (c) IgM identified, it is usually acute infection. Core antigen itself usually is observed in the asymptomatic window period but then wanes by the time symptoms appear, making detection difficult and it is not generally tested for. During chronic infection, HBs with or without detectable HBe antigen is observed, and generally, anti-HBs antibody is not detected. This patient represents a chronic infection that was likely under immune control before the immune system was suppressed by the chemotherapy and the infection reactivated.

A, B Individuals who are HBs and HBe antigen positive are in an active infection stage, and if they have HB core (c) IgM identified, it is usually acute infection.

D Those who have been infected but had resolution of their infection would have both HBs IgG and HBc antibody.

E Vaccinated individuals have detectable anti-HBs IgG as a marker but have no other positive serologies and no detectable viral DNA.

2. Correct: Cirrhosis (B)

The long-term consequence of HBV reactivation in individuals with suppressed immune systems due to chemotherapy is decreased liver function. Untreated chronic HBV infection can lead to development of cirrhosis in 5 to 20% of individuals over a 5-year period. This is exacerbated by viral reactivation. Of those with cirrhosis, 5 to 30% have a cumulative risk of developing hepatocarcinoma. While cirrhosis of the liver in many cases is observed in long-term chronic infection, thereby making hepatocellular carcinoma a more proximal event, the transient elastography results indicate that cirrhosis in not yet appearing in this case. Transient elastography is a noninvasive determination of liver stiffness by measuring the shear wave velocity emanating from an ultrasound probe as it passes through the liver.

A Atherosclerosis is not common with HBV infections.

C Of those with cirrhosis, 5 to 30% have a cumulative risk of developing hepatocarcinoma. This patient has not yet developed cirrhosis.

D Fulminant renal failure alone is not common with HBV infection but could be a secondary result of progression of the disease.

E Fulminant liver failure would likely follow the development of cirrhosis.

3. Correct: Prophylaxis with lamivudine (C)

All patients undergoing cancer treatment should be prescreened for any number of diseases which can reactivate during the treatment of cancer with immunosuppressive drugs. Among these is HBV. Unfortunately, the adoption of such screening is poor among oncologists and two large retrospective studies have shown a very poor compliance with such screening. If it were known that the patient was chronically infected with HBV before treatment, then one of two approaches could have been taken: monitor for activation of HBV by serial viral loads and treat if needed or prophylax with appropriate therapy such as lamivudine, entecavir, or tenofovir. This has been shown to be more than 80% effective in preventing reactivation.

A While avoiding alcohol is beneficial, it will not prevent a flare of the infection.

B The use of immunoglobulin has no role for this patient due to the chronic state of the infection.

D Vaccination, while very effective at preventing initial HBV infection, has no role here due to the chronic state of the infection.

E There is a proven preventative strategy and it is prophylaxis with lamivudine.

4. Correct: Reverse transcriptase (D)

The genome of HBV encodes for a polymerase that has reverse transcriptase activity. Current therapies that target viral replication are nucleos(t)ide analog inhibitors and interferon. HBV is not known to possess the remaining enzymes.

A A helicase is responsible for the separation of double-stranded DNA or RNA strands to assist in gaining access to replication machinery. An example virus that contains a helicase is HCV.

B An integrase is responsible for integration of viral nucleic acid into the host genome as in the case for retrovirus replication.

C A protease enzyme cleaves amino acid sequences by hydrolyzing peptide bonds.

E Thymidine kinase is a phosphotransferase that is available in most living cells and in some viruses such as herpes simplex virus (HSV). It functions to incorporate thymidine into growing DNA chains.

5. Correct: Tenofovir (E)

While data on the effectiveness of treatment in patients with reactivated HBV in chemotherapy are still not clear, it is agreed that treatment is appropriate. Tenofovir is a reasonable choice and does not have the same level of development of resistance that lamivudine has.

A Immunoglobulin is not an effective treatment for reactivated HBV due to the fact that it is a chronic infection.

B Development of resistance to lamivudine is common when used as a single agent and therefore it is discouraged.

C Ledipasvir/sofosbuvir is a treatment for HCV not HBV.

D This patient is not yet at the stage where he would need a liver transplant.

Keywords: Hepatitis, bloodborne pathogen, HBV, blood, alcoholic

Case 20

Adult Female with Epigastric Pain after Eating

A 33-year-old female presents with mid-epigastric pain. She states that normally the pain begins about 1 hour after eating and that the composition of her meal does not seem to impact the pain. She had been previously treated for duodenal ulcers, but her symptoms re-occurred even after treatment with antacids. The remainder of her medical history is unremarkable other than a recent upper respiratory illness for which she received azithromycin. Physical examination reveals that the patient is afebrile. The patient submitted stool for culture, ova and parasite examination, and examination for occult blood. A complete blood count was also performed. Laboratory findings indicate that the patient's stool samples are positive for occult blood, but ova and parasite examination was negative. The complete blood count was within the normal limits. An esophageal gastroduodenoscopy is performed, and a biopsy specimen is obtained. Microscopic examination of the biopsy is shown in the figure below. In addition, the biopsy tests positive for urease.

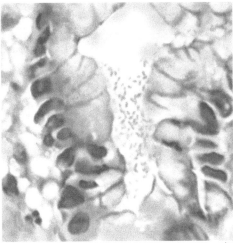

Image courtesy: Lisa D'Angelo

Questions

1. Which of the following organisms is the most likely causative agent?

A. *Bacillus cereus*

B. Enterotoxigenic *Escherichia coli*

C. *Helicobacter pylori*

D. *Staphylococcus aureus*

E. *Vibrio parahaemolyticus*

2. Which of the following culture conditions would be required to cultivate the most likely causative agent in the laboratory?

A. Aerobic atmosphere at 25°C

B. Aerobic atmosphere at 37°C

C. Aerobic atmosphere at 42°C

D. Microaerophilic atmosphere at 25°C

E. Microaerophilic atmosphere at 37°C

F. Microaerophilic atmosphere at 42°C

3. The patient comes back for a follow-up visit 6 months later. She reports that she is now 4 months pregnant. Which of the following tests could be safely used to most quickly find out if the causative agent has been eradicated?

A. Biopsy and histological staining

B. C14 breath test

C. Culture and urease test

D. Serological testing

E. Stool antigen assay

4. Which of the following is an important virulence factor that enables these microorganisms to cause ulcers?

A. Exotoxin A

B. Flagella

C. Hyaluronidase

D. Pili

E. Teichoic acid

5. At the initial presentation, which of the following would have been the most appropriate regimen for treating her illness?

A. Bismuth, metronidazole, tetracycline, and omeprazole

B. Amoxicillin, clarithromycin, and omeprazole

C. Clarithromycin, metronidazole, and omeprazole

D. Amoxicillin, clarithromycin, and metronidazole

E. High-dose omeprazole and ranitidine

Answers and Explanations

1. Correct: *Helicobacter pylori* (C)

This case describes a patient with clinical signs and symptoms of a *Helicobacter pylori* infection. She has mid-epigastric pain after eating a meal, and the symptoms do not resolve with antacid treatment. The biopsy tests positive for urease, which is a major virulence factor of *H. pylori*.

A, B, D *Bacillus cereus,* enterotoxigenic *Escherichia coli,* and *Staphylococcus aureus* are all causative agents of food poisoning, and symptoms are associated with a specific contaminated food source (which is not described in this case), therefore those three answer choices are incorrect.

E *Vibrio parahaemolyticus* infections are associated with contaminated seafood ingestion, which is not described in this case, and so *V. parahaemolyticus* is an incorrect answer.

2. Correct: Microaerophilic atmosphere at 37°C (E)

The causative agent is *H. pylori*. These bacteria may be cultured in vitro on either sheep's blood agar or selective media (e.g., Skirrow's media) in a 5% oxygen atmosphere (microaerophilic conditions) at 37°C. Colonies may take up to 7 days to become visible, so culture is not recommended in most cases.

A, B, C These bacteria require the microaerophilic conditions for optimal growth, so aerobic atmospheric conditions will result in slower growth, therefore answer choices A, B, and C are incorrect.

D, F As with most bacterial human pathogens, growth is optimal at normal human body temperature (37°C), therefore answer choices D and F are also incorrect.

3. Correct: Stool antigen assay (E)

This question is asking which diagnostic test can be used during pregnancy and give the results most quickly. With one exception, all tests listed may be safely used during pregnancy. Of all the tests listed, the stool antigen test is commonly available, the most rapid, and the most cost-effective.

A, B, C, D The urea breath test (B) uses a labeled carbon on urea which is ingested by the patient. If *H. pylori* is present, the urease enzyme that is produced will hydrolyze the urea to produce labeled CO_2 and ammonia. The labeled CO_2 can be detected by breath samples (noninvasive). The urea can be labeled with either radioactive ^{14}C or nonradioactive ^{13}C. The radioactive ^{14}C is not recommended for young children or pregnant women. The ^{13}C urea breath test is safe for both populations; however, it is not commonly available and rarely used in clinical practice. The diagnostic tests that would be the least invasive are the breath test (B) and the stool antigen assay (E) as neither would require removal of tissue or blood from the patient.

4. Correct: Flagella (B)

The causative agent is *H. pylori*. This microorganism produces many major virulence factors which allow colonization of the mucosal layer of the gastrointestinal epithelium. These virulence factors include urease production for producing a microenvironment of pH neutrality, proteases, and mucinases to allow penetration into the mucosal layer, flagella for motility, and adhesins. Flagella is the best answer choice of the options listed.

A Exotoxin A is an ADP-ribosylating toxin produced by *Pseudomonas aeruginosa* and is therefore incorrect.

C Hyaluronidase is a degradative enzyme produced by some strains of *S. aureus, Streptococcus pyogenes,* and *Clostridium perfringens* to break down host tissue during infection.

D Pili are used by many bacteria for adherence, but there is no evidence that *H. pylori* use pili for adherence to the gastrointestinal epithelia.

E Teichoic acid is a major component of the gram-positive cell wall and serves as a virulence factor for most gram-positive bacteria. However, *H. pylori* are gram-negative bacilli and therefore do not contain teichoic acid in the cell wall.

5. Correct: Bismuth, metronidazole, tetracycline, and omeprazole (A)

When treating *H. pylori*, a combination of therapies is always needed, and there are several choices. Clarithromycin is a preferred agent, but there are significant risks of resistance in *H. pylori*. Current guidelines for deciding the most appropriate treatment suggest first determining if local rates of resistance are known to be over 15% or success of eradication in the area with clarithromycin-based regimens are less than or equal to 85%. In addition, any recent exposure to macrolide antibiotics should be considered a risk of resistance, and this patient received azithromycin recently. Once clarithromycin is eliminated from the choices, the most appropriate regimen is the quadruple bismuth-based therapy which includes bismuth, metronidazole, tetracycline, and a proton pump inhibitor (PPI) such as omeprazole.

B, C These are other regimens when clarithromycin can be used.

D This option is incorrect as all regimens include a PPI.

E This is incorrect as no regimen omits antibiotics.

Keywords: Gastric ulcer, *Helicobacter pylori*, urease, flagella, bismuth

Case 21

Elderly Female with Fever and Flank Pain

A 77-year-old female presents to her primary care physician with a fever, chills, flank pain, and cloudy, foul-smelling urine. She has a past medical history of renal calculi and recurrent urinary tract infections (UTIs). Physical examination reveals a slightly anxious woman with a temperature of 38.3°C and percussion tenderness over the right flank. A urine dipstick is done in the office which reveals a urine pH of 8.2, + white blood cells (WBCs), 2+ bacteria, 3+ leukocyte esterase, and + nitrites. Her urine is sent to the microbiology laboratory for formal urinalysis, Gram stain, and culture. The patient is admitted to the hospital and an abdominal computed tomography (CT) with stone protocol is obtained. The formal urine analysis with microscopy identifies more than 100 WBC, 5 to 50 red blood cells (RBCs), and 4+ bacteria. The abdominal CT shows multiple stones in the right renal pelvis but none are obstructing. After 24 hours, the urine culture grows non–lactose-fermenting, indole-positive, urease-positive organisms. The Gram stain of the causative agent is shown in following figure.

Image courtesy: Lisa D'Angelo

Questions

1. Which of the following organisms is the most likely causative agent?

A. *Citrobacter freundii*

B. *Escherichia coli*

C. *Proteus mirabilis*

D. *Pseudomonas aeruginosa*

E. *Staphylococcus saprophyticus*

2. Which of the following describes an important virulence factor produced by the causative agent?

A. Exotoxin A

B. Flagella

C. Immunoglobulin A (IgA) protease

D. M protein

E. P-pili

3. Which of the following bacterial products from the causative agent are important for the change in pH observed in this patient's urine?

A. Flagella

B. Lipopolysaccharide

C. Peptidoglycan

D. P-fimbriae

E. Urease

4. Which of the following bacterial growth media would have been used to demonstrate that the most likely causative agent is lactose negative?

A. Blood agar

B. MacConkey's agar

C. Nutrient agar

D. Sabouraud's agar

E. Tellurite agar

5. The patient is started on ampicillin, and sensitivities reveal that the organism is sensitive to ampicillin. However, after 72 hours the patient continues to worsen, with high fever, continued flank pain, and shaking chills. Which of the following is the most likely reason for this patient's clinical decline?

A. Infected stones are not treated by antibiotics and must always be removed via cystoscopy.

B. This is not truly a UTI but rather renal colic.

C. The organism has acquired a plasmid-borne OMP2B efflux pump which is making the ceftriaxone useless.

D. The organism is not actually what was identified but is actually *Acinetobacter* which is biochemically indistinguishable from the pathogen which was identified.

E. The organism has an inducible *ampC* gene that has been activated in the presence of ampicillin and is now resistant.

Answers and Explanations

1. Correct: *Proteus mirabilis* (C)

The case describes a *Proteus* spp. infection, and all answers are organisms that may be associated with UTIs and so all are plausible answers in the absence of the microbiology laboratory results. *Proteus mirabilis* are gram-negative bacilli, lactose nonfermenters, and urease positive. Infections are associated with urinary stones.
A *Citrobacter freundii* are lactose positive and therefore incorrect.
B *Escherichia coli* are lactose positive and therefore incorrect.
D *Pseudomonas aeruginosa* is a lactose nonfermenter but is urease negative and therefore incorrect.
E *Staphylococcus saprophyticus* is gram-positive and therefore incorrect.

2. Correct: Flagella (B)

Proteus spp. are one of the most motile of the pathogenic bacteria. Flagella are peritrichous, meaning that they surround the bacterial cell (i.e., on all sides), leading to the swarming motility of this genus.
A Exotoxin A is produced by *P. aeruginosa*.
C IgA protease is produced by *Haemophilus influenzae*, *Neisseria* spp., and *Streptococcus pneumoniae*. Some species of *Proteus* also produce IgA protease, but this virulence factor is not as important as the flagella and is therefore not the best answer of those listed.
D M protein is important for *Streptococcus pyogenes* virulence.
E P-pili are important for adherence of uropathogenic strains of *E. coli* (UPEC). Proteus spp. also utilize at least four types of pili for adherence to the urinary tract, but the *Proteus* spp. pili are not termed P-pili.

3. Correct: Urease (E)

Urease is produced by *Proteus* spp. Urease causes an alkalinization of the urine pH (the patient in this case has a high urine pH of 8.2). Urease hydrolyzes urea to form ammonia and carbon dioxide. The resulting ammonia combines with hydrogen ions to form ammonium which causes an increase in the urine pH. This promotes struvite (magnesium ammonium phosphate or triple phosphate) crystals and urinary stone formation.
A, B, C, D None of the other options will result in a pH change.

4. Correct: MacConkey's agar (B)

MacConkey's agar is selective and differential. Lactose is present in the media, as is a pH indicator. Micro-organisms that are able to utilize the lactose (such as *E. coli*) will produce acidic end products, thereby causing the pH indicator to change the media color to bright pink. Growth of non–lactose fermenters (such as the causative agent in this case, *P. mirabilis*) will not result in a color change on the media.
A Blood agar is a rich medium that is not differential.
C Nutrient agar is a rich medium that is not differential.
D Sabouraud's agar is a rich medium used to cultivate many fungal organisms.
E Tellurite agar is used to isolate *Corynebacterium* spp. including *Corynebacterium diphtheriae*.

5. Correct: The organism has an inducible *ampC* gene that has been activated in the presence of ampicillin and is now resistant (E)

Proteus is one of the SPICE organisms which stands for *Serratia*, *Providencia*, indole-positive *Proteus*, *Citrobacter*, and *Enterobacter*. These organisms frequently carry inducible *ampC* beta-lactamases that render most beta-lactams inactive. The drug of choice for these organisms are non–beta-lactam antibiotics or carbapenems. Cefepime in particular is a weak inducer of *ampC* in these organisms and is fairly resistant to the activity of *ampC* beta-lactamases and may be usable.
A While infected stones may require a longer treatment to resolve and may ultimately need to be removed, a patient with infected stones should improve with antibiotics.

B Renal colic could give the pain but should not give continued clinical decline and high fevers. In addition, the CT revealed no obstructing stones.

C Efflux pumps are generally endogenous and are either upregulated or derepressed to give high-level resistance. While they can be plasmid borne, this is not the common scenario in this example.

D *Acinetobacter* and *Proteus* are both easily separated in the clinical microbiology laboratory by standard biochemical testing.

Keywords: *Proteus* spp., urinary tract, urease, motility, flagella, carbapenems, *ampC*

Case 22

Adult Male with Rash

A 39-year-old homosexual male presents to his primary care physician with a non-itchy maculopapular rash on his arms and legs and on the palms of his hands (see figure below). He reports fatigue but no other symptoms. Physical examination identified generalized lymphadenopathy and a temperature of 36.8°C. Alanine aminotransferase level was 332 IU/L and the aspartate aminotransferase level was 187 IU/L. Sexual history includes oral sex with multiple partners over the past year and infrequent condom use. An HIV point-of-care rapid test result at the time of presentation was negative.

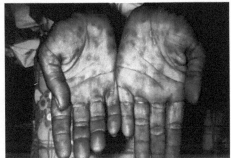

Image courtesy: CDC/ Susan Lindsley

Questions

1. Which of the following organisms is most likely responsible for this condition?

A. *Borrelia burgdorferi*

B. *Rickettsia rickettsii*

C. *Streptococcus pyogenes*

D. *Treponema pallidum*

E. Varicella-zoster virus

2. Which of the following tests is normally conducted first to aid in the screening for this agent?

A. Blood smear with darkfield microscopy

B. Skin biopsy with culture

C. Gram stain of skin scraping

D. Rapid plasma reagin (RPR)

E. Fluorescent treponemal antibody

3. What stage of the illness resulted in these symptoms?

A. Early latent

B. Late latent

C. Primary

D. Secondary

E. Tertiary

4. Another disease credited to a subspecies of this organism is transmitted by nonsexual human-to-human contact and is seen in more tropical locales. Which of the following diseases is most likely described here?

A. Haverhill fever

B. Carrion's disease

C. Tropical anhidrotic asthenia

D. Bacillary peliosis

E. Yaws

5. The patient undergoes treatment with an injection and several hours later develops fever, chills, shakes, flushing, rapid heart rate, a drop in blood pressure, muscle pain, and his rash flares and appears angrier looking. Which of the following best describes the cause of this patient's new symptoms?

A. An anaphylactic reaction

B. An Arthus reaction

C. A Jarisch–Herxheimer reaction

D. A sepsis reaction

E. A Wassermann reaction

Answers and Explanations

1. Correct: *Treponema pallidum* (D)

Given the patient history and symptoms, syphilis seems the most likely cause in this case. There is a current rise in the number of syphilis cases in men who have sex with men in those who are coinfected with HIV and those who are not. The etiology of syphilis is the bacterium *Treponema pallidum*. *Treponema* spp. are spirochetes that are gram-negative in structure but cannot be Gram stained due to the thin diameter. Darkfield microscopy is appropriate for visualization of these thin bacteria. *T. pallidum* are sexually transmitted but may also be transmitted vertically from mother to child. Syphilis is one of the TORCH infections leading to congenital anomalies in children. Syphilis is in the other (O) category along with varicella, mumps, parvovirus, HIV, and now zika virus; the others being toxoplasmosis (T), rubella (R), cytomegalovirus (C), and herpes simplex (H).

A The other organisms listed as answer choices cause rash-type symptoms, but the rash often presents in a different manner. For example, *Borrelia burgdorferi* are the causative agents of Lyme disease and are transmitted via arthropod vectors. The typical rash is described as a "bull's eye" and tends to expand outward from the site of the tick bite.
B *Rickettsia rickettsii* cause Rocky Mountain spotted fever (RMSF) and are also transmitted via arthropod vectors. The RMSF rash also tends to be non-itchy; however, it usually appears on the wrists and ankles first and then spreads in both directions.
C *Streptococcus pyogenes* or group A *Streptococcus* (GAS) causes many types of syndromes, some of which are associated with rash (i.e., scarlet fever).
E The varicella-zoster virus is the causative agent of chickenpox.

2. Correct: Rapid plasma reagin (RPR) (D)

Initial testing for syphilis uses non-*Treponema*–specific tests such as the Venereal Disease Research Laboratory (VDRL) test that detects antibodies produced in response to infection with *T. pallidum*. However, there are several other infections that can result in a false-positive test result. An additional nonspecific test used for screening is the RPR test. Both of these tests have higher specificity when applied in the earlier stages of infection. Positive test results require confirmatory testing with *Treponema*-specific tests such as the *T. pallidum* particle agglutination test under the current testing algorithms or the fluorescent treponemal antibody test. In some testing sites, a reverse algorithm is being applied where *Treponema*-specific testing is done by automated enzyme immunoassay. Positive tests are then reflexed to RPR testing to determine staging. At present, rapid point-of-care *Treponema* tests are being evaluated for use in diagnostic algorithms.

A Darkfield microscopy is a way of visualizing the treponemal spirochete, but it is not in common use.
B A skin biopsy and culture is not typically used for diagnosis of syphilis.
C A Gram stain of the skin would not reveal the spirochetes.
E A Fluorescent treponemal antibody test is usually done after the initial screening test for syphilis, the RPR. This is a confirmatory test for *T. pallidum*.

3. Correct: Secondary (D)

This is a case of secondary stage syphilis. Secondary syphilis is characterized often by the presence of a rash with a rough and faint reddish-brown appearance over the body, particularly on the palms of the hands and soles of the feet. Other symptoms beyond what is described in this case, such as sore throat, patchy hair loss, headache, and weight loss, may occur. Secondary syphilis is a progressive illness that occurs approximately 6 to 8 weeks after untreated primary syphilis.

A, B Resolution of symptoms of secondary syphilis will occur without treatment resulting in a latent stage infection. An untreated infection that has become latent can be undetected for several years. This patient does not have latent syphilis because the patient is symptomatic.

C Primary syphilis is predominantly characterized by a chancre that may be painless and go unnoticed.

E A small percentage of these infections may proceed to a more severe form of infection identified as tertiary or late stage syphilis. At this stage, the primary symptoms are neurological with difficulty of muscle coordination, peripheral numbness, blindness, or dementia. Damage to internal organs resulting from the infection can lead to death.

4. Correct: Yaws (E)

Yaws is a disease that appears as skin papillomas or ulcers and is caused by the *T. pallidum* subspecies *pertenue*. There are three stages to infection as in syphilis, but transmission is via nonsexual skin-to-skin contact. The secondary stages may involve bones and joints beyond the skin manifestations. In tertiary yaws, destruction of soft tissues may occur. Other diseases caused by different *T. pallidum* subspecies include *pinta* and *bejel*.

A Haverhill fever is a type of rat-bite fever caused by *Streptobacillus moniliformis*.

B Carrion's disease, also known as Oroya fever is caused by *Bartonella bacilliformis*.

C Tropical anhidrotic asthenia is another name for prickly heat.

D Bacillary peliosis is a form of *Bartonella* infection seen in HIV patients in which vascular abnormalities form in the liver.

5. Correct: *A* Jarisch–Herxheimer reaction (C)

A commonly noted reaction in patients treated for infections caused by spirochetes is the Jarisch–Herxheimer reaction. This is caused by spillage of bacterial endotoxin upon lysis of the spirochetes by antibiotics and is generally self-limiting and, while uncomfortable and can appear to be serious, is in general not a truly serious event. Severe sepsis can certainly present as described in this question, but the timing of the reaction makes it much less likely.

A Patients can certainly anaphylax to penicillin which is the treatment of choice for syphilis, but the spectrum of symptoms seen in this patient makes anaphylaxis less likely and Jarisch-Herxheimer more likely.

B An Arthus reaction is typically described in patients who receive vaccinations where they already have high levels of pre-existing antibodies; tetanus is the classic vaccine that causes Arthus reactions. It is a type III hypersensitivity reaction in which antigen-antibody complexes are formed and cause a localized vasculitis presenting with erythema, swelling, induration, and pain at the injection site and can mimic the appearance of cellulitis.

D Sepsis is when bacteria infect the blood. This rarely occurs in *T. pallidum* infections.

E A Wasserman reaction is a complement fixation test which can be used in the diagnosis of syphilis.

Keywords: Syphilis, STD, *Treponema pallidum*, rash, lymphadenopathy

Case 23 Young Female with Joint Pain

A 20-year-old female presents to her primary care physician with joint pain for the past week. She states that the joint pain seems to "move around" and that it is not always the same joint that is sore each day. Past medical history indicates that she has had no significant medical issues previously and she is up-to-date on all required vaccinations. Her family history is negative for any rheumatologic disorders. Her social history is that she is a college student who works at a local bookstore part-time, a nonsmoker, drinks alcohol on weekends, and usually gets drunk once a month at parties. She admits to occasional use of marijuana but denies any other illicit drug use. She has not travelled out of the country recently and has no animal exposures. When asked about her sexual history, she states she is not active and is a virgin; however, when questioned deeper she reveals that she regularly engages in heterosexual manual and oral sex, most often fellatio. She reports to have engaged in fellatio with multiple partners in the past 2 months. Physical examination reveals a temperature of 37°C, blood pressure of 120/75 mmHg, respiratory rate of 14 breaths/min, and pulse of 82 bpm. Her right knee, left wrist, and left ankle are all swollen and tender. Given her history, a throat swab is sent to the laboratory for Gram stain and culture. The Gram stain is shown in the figure below. A sample of synovial fluid is obtained and found to have a high white blood cell count, but a Gram stain is negative.

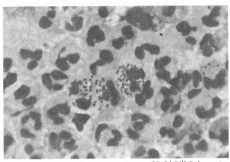

Image courtesy: CDC/ Bill Schwartz

Questions

1. Which of the following organisms is the most likely causative agent of this patient's symptoms?

A. *Chlamydia trachomatis*

B. *Haemophilus influenzae*

C. *Neisseria gonorrhoeae*

D. *Streptococcus pyogenes*

E. *Treponema pallidum*

2. Which of the following agars would be best for culture of the most likely causative agent?

A. Bordet–Gengou agar

B. Charcoal yeast agar

C. Lowenstein–Jensen agar

D. MacConkey's agar

E. Thayer–Martin agar

3. Which of the following is an important characteristic of the causative agent?

A. Inability to produce adenosine triphosphate (ATP)

B. Motility with an undulating membrane and flagella

C. Production of a triple-layered unit membrane containing sterol

D. Presence of surface pili

E. Visualization by darkfield microscopy

4. Nucleic acid amplification testing (NAAT) is performed on the patient's male partners. Which is the most appropriate sample for this testing?

A. Urethra

B. Urine

C. Throat

D. Rectum

E. NAAT is not an appropriate test in men

5. Which of the following is the most appropriate therapy for this patient?

A. Ceftriaxone 1 g IV daily for 14 days

B. Ceftriaxone 2 g IV ×1 dose

C. Azithromycin 1 g PO ×1 dose

D. Ciprofloxacin 500 mg PO twice a day for 14 days

E. Ciprofloxacin 400 mg IV twice a day for 14 days

Answers and Explanations

1. Correct: *Neisseria gonorrhoeae* (C)

Described in this case is a patient with disseminated gonorrheal infection which is caused by *Neisseria gonorrhoeae*. The migratory joint pain is a classic sign of disseminated gonococcal infection and can be seen in purulent arthritis or the "arthritis–dermatitis syndrome," which generally has a rash and inflammation of the tendons as well. *Neisseria* spp. are intracellular gram-negative diplococci as shown in the figure. The only other pathogenic *Neisseria* species are *Neisseria meningitidis*, which does not cause this syndrome. *N. gonorrhoeae* are strict human pathogens with no known animal reservoir. With disseminated gonorrheal infection there is generally an initial infection of the mucous membranes. This patient was likely infected by the pathogen while performing oral sex on a male partner who was infected with *N. gonorrhoeae*, and thus the organism can usually be found in the throat. Despite having a purulent arthritis, the organism is often not isolated from the joints. Infection by *N. gonorrhoeae* in a man typically manifests as dysuria, penile discharge, and painful or swollen testes.
A *Chlamydia trachomatis* is also a sexually transmitted infection; however, they cannot be visualized by Gram stain and do not usually cause sore throat or joint pain.
B *Haemophilus influenzae* is a causative agent of sore throat; however joint pain is rarely a symptom of infection. Furthermore, *H. influenzae* are gram-negative bacilli that are not normally intracellular.
D *Streptococcus pyogenes* is the causative agent of strep throat. *S. pyogenes* (or group A *Streptococcus* [GAS]) do not normally cause joint pain and are gram-positive cocci.
E *Treponema pallidum* is the causative agent of syphilis and is a spirochete that is normally visualized by darkfield microscopy.

2. Correct: Thayer–Martin agar (E)

This case describes a patient with joint pain and a sore throat caused by *N. gonorrhoeae*. These organisms are fastidious and are unable to grow on routine blood agar without the presence of X (hemin) and V (nicotinamide adenine dinucleotide [NAD]) factors. Thayer–Martin agar is used to culture *Neisseria* species as it also contains antibiotics to prevent the overgrowth of other organisms. Culture is becoming increasingly important because it allows for antibiotic susceptibility data to be obtained.
A Bordet-Gengou agar is used for culturing *Bordetella pertussis*, the causative agent of whooping cough.
B Charcoal yeast agar is used for the isolation of *Legionella pneumophila*.
C Lowenstein-Jensen agar is the media used for the growth of mycobacterial species such as *Mycobacterium tuberculosis*, the causative agent of tuberculosis (TB).
D MacConkey's agar is a selective and differential agar is used for enteric gram-negative bacilli.

3. Correct: Presence of surface pili (D)

This case describes a patient with gonococcal-associated joint pain due to a disseminated infection by *N. gonorrhoeae*. These pathogens are facultative intracellular gram-negative diplococci, as can be seen in the figure. The first stage of infection by this pathogen following entry into the body is attachment to host epithelial cells. The adhesins for initial attachment are type IV pili, Opa proteins (opacity-associated proteins), and genus-specific lipooligosaccharide (LOS). In addition to adhesion to host cells, pili are used for DNA transfer, often leading to transfer of antibiotic resistance traits between strains.
A *N. gonorrhoeae* are able to produce ATP, unlike *C. trachomatis*, which has the inability to produce ATP.
B *Trichomonas vaginalis* are protozoa that are motile by the use of undulating membranes and flagella.
C Fungi produce triple-layered unit membranes that contain sterol.
E *T. pallidum*, the causative agent of syphilis is normally visualized by darkfield microscopy due to the thinness of the bacterial spirochetes.

93

4. Correct: Urine (B)

This case describes a patient with a gonococcal pharyngeal infection that she obtained while engaging in oral sex with a partner who was presumably infected with *N. gonorrhoeae*. If possible, NAAT would be performed on the patient's partners to confirm the diagnosis and prevent further transmission of the pathogen. NAAT is an accurate molecular test with high sensitivity and specificity for both genital and extragenital infections. NAAT has the advantage of giving accurate results more rapidly than cultures. The biggest disadvantage of NAAT is that antibiotic resistance/sensitivity data cannot be determined (and therefore possible options for treatment are also not given with NAAT).

A, C, D NAAT can be used with all the specimens listed in this question, however, given that the patient likely acquired the infection from fellatio, the partner would most likely have a genital infection. Both a urethral swab and urine can be used for NAAT testing, but in men they have equal sensitivity, and a urethral swab is fairly invasive and painful, thus urine is considered the appropriate specimen.

E NAAT is appropriate for all sexual partners, regardless of gender.

5. Correct: Ceftriaxone 1 g IV daily for 14 days (A)

Currently, ceftriaxone is considered the first-line therapy for the treatment of disseminated gonorrheal infection. When treating purulent arthritis, current guidelines suggest 1 g IV daily for 7 to 14 days.

B A single dose of ceftriaxone is inappropriate for management of purulent arthritis as a longer duration is necessary to clear the infection.

C A single dose of azithromycin is inappropriate for the management of purulent arthritis.

D, E Ciprofloxacin may work but is no longer considered first line due to high levels of resistance. It would not be appropriate to hold off therapy until antibiotic susceptibility can be obtained from culture. Resistance to ceftriaxone is a rising problem and the Centers for Disease Control and Prevention (CDC) has declared it one of three urgent threats due to resistance.

Keywords: *Neisseria gonorrhoeae*, sexually transmitted infection, Thayer-Martin, type IV pili, lipooligosaccharide (LOS), antibiotic resistance, nucleic acid amplification testing, ceftriaxone

Case 24

Teenager with Syncopy

A 16-year-old adolescent male is brought to the emergency department in the evening after a syncopal episode. He had been in a fistfight at school 2 days earlier which resulted in a nosebleed, which he self-treated by packing his nostrils with gauze. Upon questioning, the patient stated that he gets nosebleeds frequently and has often used nasal packing for treatment with no issues. Past medical history indicates that the patient is an otherwise healthy male with no previous serious illnesses or surgeries. He is up-to-date on all routine vaccinations. Physical examination reveals an ill-appearing and somewhat confused young man with a diffuse erythematous rash on his trunk and extremities. Examination of the nose indicates the presence of the nasal packing which is removed without issue. No further bleeding occurs at the patient's nose, and palpation of the area does not elicit pain. The remainder of the examination of the head reveals a swollen, bumpy tongue (see figure below) and significant redness of the conjunctiva. The patient's temperature is 39.5°C, respiratory rate (RR) is 25 breaths/min, heart rate (HR) is 136 bpm, and BP is 89/50 mmHg. The patient vomited several times in the waiting room as well as during the physical examination. The patient notes diffuse muscle aches. STAT laboratories are sent and reveal a white blood cell (WBC) count of 50,000/uL, platelets of 75,000/uL, his blood urea nitrogen (BUN) is 45 and his creatinine is 4.7, his alanine aminotransferase (ALT) is 345 and his aspartate aminotransferase (AST) is 378; he has a total bilirubin of 1.9. His creatine phosphokinase (CPK) is 200.

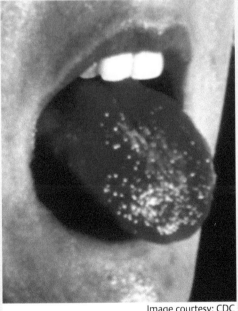

Image courtesy: CDC

Questions

1. Which of the following organisms is the most likely causative agent?

A. *Clostridium botulinum*

B. *Clostridium tetani*

C. *Rickettsia rickettsii*

D. *Staphylococcus aureus*

E. *Streptococcus pyogenes*

2. Which of the following toxins is the most likely cause of this patient's symptoms?

A. Botulinum toxin

B. Enterotoxin C

C. Shiga toxin

D. Tetanospasmin

E. Toxic shock syndrome toxin-1 (TSST-1)

3. Which of the following best describes the mode of action of the virulence factor most likely responsible for the symptoms seen in this patient?

A. ADP-ribosylation of elongation factor 2 (EF-2)

B. Cyclic adenosine monophosphate (cAMP) activity

C. Mobilization of host cell actin

D. Protease

E. Superantigen

4. Which of the following best describes the cellular morphology of the most likely causative agent?

A. Gram-negative bacilli

B. Gram-negative cocci

C. Gram-positive bacilli

D. Gram-positive cocci

E. Non–Gram-staining bacteria

5. In addition to supportive care, which of the following is the most appropriate treatment at this point in the patient's care?

A. Vancomycin + clindamycin

B. Penicillin + clindamycin

C. Vancomycin + piperacillin–tazobactam

D. Intravenous immunoglobulin (IVIg)

E. Doxycycline

Answers and Explanations

1. Correct: *Staphylococcus aureus* (D)

This patient presents with signs and symptoms of toxic shock syndrome (TSS), caused by *Staphylococcus aureus*. TSS can occur upon blood exposure to the organism (examples include childbirth, surgical wound infections, mastitis, sinusitis, osteomyelitis, cutaneous and subcutaneous lesions). Historically, TSS is associated with tampon use in a menstruating female, especially if left in the vagina for long periods of time. However, use of tampons or other packing in the nasal cavity yields similar results, as illustrated in this case. Symptoms include a fever above or equal to 38.9°C, seizures, a diffuse and red macular rash that resembles a sunburn and moves centripetally and leads to desquamation of the palms and soles, vomiting, diarrhea, confusion, and syncope. Hypotensive shock leads to organ failure, frequently involving both the kidneys and liver (as indicated by the laboratory results for this patient) at the time of diagnosis.

A *Clostridium botulinum* causes botulism, an infection that involves paralysis.

B *Clostridium tetani* causes tetanus, an infection that involves paralysis.

C *Rickettsia rickettsii* causes Rocky Mountain spotted fever (RMSF), which is often associated with a petechial rash and involves an insect bite.

E Although *S. aureus* is the causative agent of TSS, described in this case, *Streptococcus pyogenes* can also cause a toxic shock-like syndrome (TSLS). TSLS is more commonly associated with extreme pain at the site of the initial trauma (in this case, the nose), so it is less likely to be the cause of the toxic shock. In addition, TSS due to *S. aureus* is more common with nasal packing due to frequent colonization of the nares by *S. aureus*.

2. Correct: Toxic shock syndrome toxin-1 (TSST-1) (E)

This patient presents with signs and symptoms of TSS, caused by the TSST-1 produced by *S. aureus*. *S. aureus* also produces Enterotoxin C (as well as enterotoxins A, B, D, E, and H), which causes food poisoning and not the symptoms described in this case. Interestingly, there is evidence for involvement of *S. aureus* enterotoxin B and enterotoxin A in TSS; however more research is required.

A Botulinum toxin is a neurotoxin that cause flaccid paralysis and is produced by *Clostridium botulinum*.

B *S. aureus* also produced Enterotoxin C, which is associated with food poisoning, not mentioned in this case.

C Shiga toxin is produced by *Shigella* spp. and some strains of *Escherichia coli* (Shiga toxin-producing *E. coli* [STEC] strains) and causes dysentery or bloody diarrhea.

D Tetanospasmin toxin is a neurotoxin that causes spastic paralysis and is produced by *Clostridium tetani*.

3. Correct: Superantigen (E)

S. aureus exotoxins, including TSST-1, act as superantigens. During infection, the TSST-1 exotoxin is produced by *S. aureus* and acts as a superantigen to activate large numbers of host T cells in an antigen-independent manner. Superantigens bind major histocompatibility complex (MHC) class II with T-cell receptors (TCRs) of the immune system in an antigen-independent fashion, thereby activating the T cell and inducing a massive cytokine production. Activated T cells release interleukin-1 (IL-1), IL-2, tumor necrosis factor-α (TNF-α), TNF-β, and interferon-γ (INF-γ) in large quantities, which result in the symptoms of toxic shock syndrome.

A This is another typical bacterial exotoxin activity. ADP-ribosylation of EF-2 is an activity of *Pseudomonas aeruginosa* exotoxin A and also *Corynebacterium diphtheriae* toxin.

B This is another typical bacterial exotoxin activity. Vibrio cholera toxin exhibits cAMP activity

C This is another typical bacterial exotoxin activity. Many stains of *Listeria monocytogenes* as well as *Trypanosoma cruzi* produce proteins that are able to mobilize of host cell actin.

D This is another typical bacterial exotoxin activity. Tetanus and botulinum neurotoxins both act as intracellular proteases.

4. Correct: Gram-positive cocci (D)

This case describes TSS, caused by the TSST-1 produced by *S. aureus*. Although the isolation of *S. aureus* is not required for diagnosis of staphylococcal TSS, the organism can be recovered from wounds and mucosal sites in approximately 80% of patients with TSS, but only from the blood in approximately 5% of cases. *S. aureus* are gram-positive cocci that are arranged in clusters when viewed microscopically.

A *S. aureus* are not gram-negative bacilli, they are gram-positive cocci.

B *S. aureus* are not gram-negative cocci, they are gram-positive cocci.

C *S. aureus* are not gram-positive bacilli, they are gram-positive cocci.

E *S. aureus* are not non-Gram-staining bacteria, they are gram-positive cocci.

5. Correct: Vancomycin + clindamycin (A)

The treatment of TSS is first and foremost supportive care, IV fluids, pressors, intubation if needed, etc. The infection is generally treated with a combination of an antibiotic targeting the causative organism and a second antibiotic which is a protein synthesis inhibitor to stop toxin production. The most commonly used antibiotic for toxin blockade is clindamycin, however, there are reports of using other protein synthesis inhibitors such as linezolid when methicillin-resistant *S. aureus* (MRSA) is highly suspected as the cause. MRSA-based TSS has been widely reported in Japan but remains relatively rare in the United States despite the overall common nature of MRSA. While MRSA is rare as a cause of TSS, it is not unheard of, as such starting treatment with vancomycin to cover MRSA is reasonable and appropriate making choice A correct.

B Choice B would be correct if streptococcal toxic shock was suspected, but *S. aureus* is generally penicillin resistant.

C Choice C is appropriate for empiric treatment of septic shock but not toxic shock.

D IVIg is often used as a supplement for treatment of TSS which is meant to diminish the superantigen reaction and has better evidence for activity against streptococcal toxic shock. It is not meant to take the place of antibiotics and still has limited clinical evidence of efficacy.

E Doxycycline would be appropriate for Rocky Mountain spotted fever but not TSS.

Keywords: Toxic shock syndrome, TSST-1, *Staphylococcus aureus*, *Streptococcus pyogenes*, superantigen

Case 25

Adult Male with Painful Penile Ulcers

A 30-year-old male presents to a primary care physician with concerns of significantly painful swelling in the groin. The patient immigrated to the United States from Nicaragua 1 week ago. He developed painful ulcers on the penis that appeared approximately 2 weeks previously. Upon physical examination, a deep painful well-demarcated tissue ulcer of approximately 1 cm in diameter was observed on the base of his penis and two other lesions of approximately the same size were noted just proximal posterior to the glans (see figure below). There is a small amount of blood noted on his underwear. Examination of the groin reveals large, tender fluctuant swellings bilaterally in the inguinal area. An exudate from an ulcer was collected and placed on a slide for microscopic examination. Under both Gram stain and darkfield microscopy, no organisms were identified.

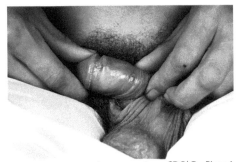

Image courtesy: CDC/ Dr. Pirozzi

Questions

1. Which of the following agents most likely is the cause of this illness?

A. *Chlamydia trachomatis*

B. *Haemophilus ducreyi*

C. Herpes simplex virus type 2 (HSV-2)

D. *Klebsiella granulomatis*

E. *Treponema pallidum*

2. Which of the following are required for growth of this organism in culture?

A. Cholic acid

B. Hemin

C. Human foreskin fibroblasts

D. Nicotinamide adenine dinucleotide

E. Ornithine

3. Which of the following is accepted as the most probable evidence of a case of this disease?

A. At least one painful genital ulcer, nonreactive rapid plasma reagin (RPR), negative HSV polymerase chain reaction (PCR)

B. Multiple painful genital ulcers at the base of the glans, nonreactive RPR, negative Gram stain

C. At least one painful genital ulcer, nonreactive RPR, negative Tzanck smear

D. Multiple painful genital ulcers at the base of the glans, nonreactive RPR, noted bleeding from the ulcers

E. At least one painful genital ulcer, nonreactive RPR, positive CLIA-verified PCR test

4. Which of the following is considered the first-line treatment for this infection?

A. Azithromycin

B. Doxycycline

C. Gentamicin

D. Penicillin

E. Trimethoprim–sulfamethoxazole

5. What is the most appropriate treatment for the groin lesions in addition to the antibiotics?

A. No additional treatment is needed; they will resolve with antibiotic therapy

B. Incision and drainage

C. Wide area resection of the lesion

D. Injection of the same antibiotic into the lesion

E. Hot compresses to the area until they drain spontaneously

Answers and Explanations

1. Correct: *Haemophilus ducrey* (B)

This is a case of chancroid due to *Haemophilus ducreyi* infection. *H. ducreyi* is rarely seen in the United States but is an important pathogen globally with higher incidence in underdeveloped countries of Africa, Latin America, and the Caribbean. Given the nationality and age of the patient, sexually transmitted chancroid should be considered.

A *Chlamydia trachomatis* infection often produces small ulcerative lesions, but these are usually accompanied by urethral discharge, not seen in this case.

C HSV usually produces small blisters without inguinal lymphadenopathy and buboes.

D *Klebsiella granulomatis* is the causative agent of granuloma inguinale, which tends to manifest as ulcerative lesions resulting from painless nodules. Lymphadenopathy is most often absent in cases of *K. granulomatous*.

E *Treponema pallidum*, the causative agent of syphilis, can produce similar lesions in the genital region during the primary stage of infection, but the negative result of dark-field microscopy would make this pathogen less likely. Furthermore, the chancre of syphilis is painless while the chancroid lesions are painful, as seen with this patient.

2. Correct: Hemin (B)

H. ducreyi is a fastidious gram-negative organism that requires hemin (X factor) for growth. A typical Gram stain is shown in the following figure. It is difficult to culture and requires a temperature not to exceed 35°C and a microaerophilic atmosphere. The organism only grows in humans and must be cultured within 4 hours on complex media.

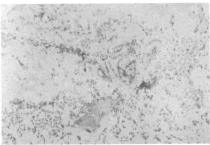

Image courtesy: CDC/ Joe Miller; Dr. N. J. Fiumara

A Cholic acid is a bile acid that has inhibitory properties on gut microflora.

C Human foreskin fibroblasts are a suitable cell for production of HSV in culture.

D Other *Haemophilus* species, such as influenzae may require additional components such as NAD (V factor). X and V factor can be used to differentiate *Haemophilus* species in culture.

E Ornithine is a metabolic product of L-arginine catabolism in *Treponema* spp.

3. Correct: At least one painful genital ulcer, nonreactive rapid plasma reagin (RPR), negative HSV polymerase chain reaction (PCR) (A)

Definitive diagnosis of *H. ducreyi* is difficult and can be made by culture of the organism on specialized media. At present, there aren't any Food and Drug Administration (FDA)-cleared molecular tests for *H. ducreyi*, but laboratory developed tests are available and, if run in a CLIA-certified laboratory, are considered definitive evidence of the infection by the Centers for Disease Control and Prevention (CDC). Because of the other pathogens that may cause ulcerations, clinical signs alone are not conclusive for diagnosis. The CDC has a definition of a probable case of chancroid which includes the following: (1) the patient has one or more painful genital ulcers; (2) the clinical presentation, appearance of genital ulcers, and, if present, regional lymphadenopathy are typical for chancroid; (3) the patient has no evidence of *T. pallidum* infection by darkfield examination of ulcer exudate or by a serologic test for syphilis performed at least 7 days after onset of ulcers; and (4) an HSV PCR test or HSV culture performed on the ulcer exudate is negative.

B, C, D, E In regard to the first requirement, at least one painful genital ulcer is needed which eliminates choices B and D. In regard to the second requirement, all of the answers ask for a typical appearance and clinical presentation and none discussed the buboes/lymphadenopathy which this patient does have. In regard to the third requirement, all of the answers ask for a negative test for syphilis (RPR). In regard to the last requirement, there must be a negative PCR or culture test for HSV; while the Tzanck smear is a test for HSV, it does not qualify under this definition eliminating choice C. Choice E asks for a positive PCR test which per the CDC would be a definitive case even though not FDA approved. This leaves choice A as the answer which meets all the criteria.

4. Correct: Azithromycin (A)

Azithromycin as a single 1 g dose is considered first line for treating chancroid. Other recommended regimens include ceftriaxone as a single 250 mg intramuscular (IM) dose, ciprofloxacin 500 mg PO BID for 3 days, and erythromycin 500 mg PO TID for 7 days. The single oral dose makes Azithromycin preferred among these regimens.

Both ciprofloxacin and erythromycin are also less favored due to known resistance seen worldwide which makes their use difficult since culture and resistance testing are not routinely performed.

B, C, D, E The other antibiotics listed as choices are not used to treat chancroid.

5. Correct: Incision and drainage (B)

Fluctuant buboes from chancroid generally require drainage which can be accomplished by standard incision and drainage or needle aspiration. Needle aspiration due to the more limited amount drained often needs to be repeated. Without drainage buboes may go on to spontaneously drain and form fistulous tracks.

A Treatment by incision and drainage is required for this infection.

C There is no need for wide area resection such as would be used in necrotizing fasciitis.

D There is no need for injection of antibiotic directly into a bubo.

E Bringing about spontaneous drainage is exactly what we try to avoid by performing an incision and drainage to reduce the chance of forming fistula. Hot compresses are often used to bring a boil to the head but would not be effective in draining a bubo.

Keywords: Buboes, chancroid, *Haemophilus ducreyi*, sexually transmitted infection

Case 26

Adult Male with Back Pain

A 38-year-old male immigrant from Africa presents to the emergency department with mid-back pain which came on slowly. He states that the back pain started about a month ago and has increased in severity since he first noticed it. Past medical history reveals that the patient is generally healthy but recalls being hospitalized once as a teenager. He does not recall whether he was diagnosed with a specific illness at that time. He does remember that he received several medications and that the medication the doctor had given him caused his tears to turn orange. He recalls having a full recovery and has not required hospitalization since that time. He reports that he has "colds" occasionally (as most people do), but otherwise he feels that he has been quite healthy until now.

He immigrated to the United States shortly after his experience in the hospital in Africa and has not traveled outside the United States since. He has no unusual exposures other than his coming from Africa. He is HIV negative and has no history of incarceration or exposure to the health care system. Physical examination reveals an uncomfortable man with no specific findings except pain on palpation of his spine in the thoracic region. His vitals are all within normal limits. Radiography of the chest shows a paraspinal mass at T7–T8. A biopsy of the mass is performed by interventional radiology and sent for culture and staining, one of which reveals the organism shown in the figure below.

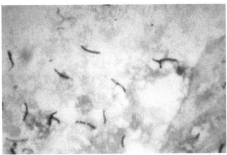

Image courtesy: CDC/ Dr. George P. Kubica

Questions

1. Which of the following is the most likely special stain that was used to identify the causative organism?

A. Calcofluor white

B. Brown and Brenn

C. Malachite green

D. Acridine orange

E. Auramine–rhodamine

2. For the most likely pathogen, which agar would be used for isolation?

A. Chocolate agar

B. Eaton's agar

C. Löffler's medium

D. Löwenstein–Jensen agar

E. Thayer–Martin media

3. Which cells were responsible for initially containing this infection?

A. CD4+ T lymphocytes and B lymphocytes

B. CD4+ T lymphocytes and macrophages

C. CD4+ T lymphocytes and natural killer (NK) cells

D. CD4+ T lymphocytes and neutrophils

E. CD8+ T lymphocytes and B lymphocytes

F. NK cells and macrophages

4. Which of the following best describes the outer surface of the most likely causative agent?

A. Lipid bilayer containing ergosterols

B. Mycolic acid glycolipids

C. Protein capsule

D. Thick peptidoglycan layer

E. Thin peptidoglycan layer plus an outer membrane

5. Given the presentation and history of this patient, what is the most appropriate initial therapy?

A. Isoniazid, rifampin, pyrazinamide, moxifloxacin, streptomycin

B. Isoniazid, rifampin, pyrazinamide, moxifloxacin, bedaquiline

C. Isoniazid, rifampin, ethambutol, pyrazinamide

D. Isoniazid, rifampin, ethambutol

E. Isoniazid and rifampin

Answers and Explanations

1. Correct: Auramine–rhodamine (E)

The patient has a tuberculosis reactivation infection. Tuberculosis is caused by *Mycobacterium tuberculosis*. *M. tuberculosis* stain red with an acid-fast stain (as shown in the figure) and are often described as acid-fast bacilli (AFB). This patient was infected with the bacteria at an earlier date and the infection is reactivated with the symptoms described. The patient had been diagnosed with tuberculosis previously and had been prescribed rifampin, which can cause orange secretions. Typical symptoms of reactivation tuberculosis begin insidiously and develop over weeks or months before diagnosis. Most patients present with cough, weight loss, fever, night sweats, and fatigue. Mycobacteria are visualized using acid-fast stains. The most common stains used are carbol fuchsin and Auramine–rhodamine. Laboratories more frequently use Auramine–rhodamine as it can be seen using florescence microscopy and is more sensitive than carbol fuchsin which is visualized using light microscopy.

A, B, C, D Calcofluor white is used for fungal visualization. Brown and Brenn is a tissue stain. Malachite green is used for the bacterial endospore stain. Acridine orange stains nucleic acids.

2. Correct: Löwenstein–Jensen agar (D)

The patient described here is suffering from tuberculosis with typical symptoms of back pain, fever, weight loss, and night sweats. *M. tuberculosis* is not often cultured in the laboratory due to the fact that growth is extremely slow, taking 3 to 4 weeks for growth. The organisms do not grow on routine culture media and must be grown on media with albumin such as Löwenstein–Jensen agar, which is mint green in color. Alternatively, the organism can be cultivated in potato- and egg-based media, such as Middlebrook 7H10 or 7H11.

A Chocolate agar would be used to grow fastidious organisms such as *Haemophilus influenzae*.
B Eaton's agar is used for the growth of *Mycoplasma pneumoniae*.
C Löffler's medium is used for the growth of *Corynebacterium diphtheriae*.
E Thayer–Martin media is utilized for isolation of *Neisseria gonorrhoeae*.

3. Correct: CD4+ T lymphocytes and macrophages (B)

Pulmonary tuberculosis infections are controlled or contained within caseous granulomas. It is primarily CD4+ T lymphocytes (T-helper lymphocytes) and macrophages of the immune system that are responsible for initially containing the infection and allowing the formation of the granulomas. Upon entry into the lungs, *M. tuberculosis* are taken up by alveolar macrophages and are able to survive intracellularly within the phagosomes of those macrophages. Upon activation, the alveolar macrophages also produce cytokines and chemokines that attract other phagocytic cells (neutrophils, monocytes, and further alveolar macrophages) to the site of infection. Following an initial infection, the patient will become asymptomatic due to the action of the CD4+ T lymphocytes and the macrophages.

A, C, D, E, F B lymphocytes, NK cells, and neutrophils are not believed to be involved with containing tuberculosis infections.

4. Correct: Mycolic acid glycolipids (B)

The outer surface of *Mycobacterium* species is composed of mycolic acid glycolipids and waxy-like substances that are impermeable to most routine staining procedures. The cell envelope is a distinguishing feature of the *Mycobacterium* genus. The cell wall components cause the organism to resist the destaining with acid-alcohol step during the Ziehl–Neelsen stain, and thus stain acid-fast positive.

A, C, D, E A lipid bilayer containing ergosterols describes a typical fungal cell envelope. A protein capsule is produced by *Bacillus anthracis*; however, most bacterial capsules are composed of polysaccharides.

Gram-positive organisms produce a thick peptidoglycan layer, which is the basis for the Gram stain procedure. Gram-negative organisms produce a thin peptidoglycan layer that is surrounded by an outer membrane that is composed of a lipid inner leaflet and an outer leaflet containing lipopolysaccharide. The relatively impermeable outer layer of *M. tuberculosis* is thought to be an important virulence factor that allows that organism to survive in the environment, form a granuloma, and survive intracellularly within alveolar macrophages.

5. Correct: Isoniazid, rifampin, pyrazinamide, moxifloxacin, streptomycin (A)

Empiric treatment of tuberculosis should include a consideration of drug resistance to help guide therapy. Empiric expanded therapy for drug-resistant strains should be considered in patients who fail treatment, who relapse after apparent cure, with known exposure to drug-resistant tuberculosis or who traveled to or resided in an area with high prevalence of drug-resistant tuberculosis. This patient was previously treated many years ago, and while this could be a new infection, the history of when he immigrated and his exposures since make this more likely a relapse. In addition, we know that he specifically received a rifamycin such as rifampin due to the history of orange tears. This makes resistance to rifampin more likely. Empiric regimens for suspected resistant tuberculosis should include isoniazid, rifampin, and pyrazinamide plus two additional drugs including a quinolone and an injectable. Choice A includes this regimen.

B, C, D, E Choice B replaced the injectable with bedaquiline which is a recently approved anti-tuberculosis drug saved for resistant tuberculosis and is generally not added empirically to preserve it as an agent of last resort. Choice C through E contain too few drugs for empiric treatment of suspected resistant tuberculosis.

Keywords: Tuberculosis, *Mycobacterium tuberculosis*, isoniazid, rifampin, pyrazinamide

Case 27

Adult Female with Vaginal Discharge

A 46-year-old female was seen by her primary care physician for symptoms of thick, odorless white–gray vaginal discharge, itching, and a burning sensation when urinating for the past 2 days. She tried to treat herself with over-the-counter topical Monistat (miconazole) but was unsuccessful. She reports that this is her sixth occurrence of similar symptoms this year and that she was previously treated with fluconazole by the urgent care clinic. The woman is recently divorced and has had two sex partners over the past year, has not used oral contraceptives and claims irregular condom use. The woman reports being in generally good health. On physical examination, all vital signs are normal. Abnormal findings on the examination include easily detachable white patches on the mucosa of the vagina with underlying erythematous bases; bilateral detachable white patches on an erythematous base were also observed on the lateral surfaces of the tongue and elsewhere on the oral mucosa; generalized lymphadenopathy was noted in the cervical, supraclavicular, and inguinal regions.

Vaginal pH was determined to be 4.5. A vaginal swab was sent for potassium hydroxide (KOH) preparation and a vaginal culture was ordered which grew an organism on yeast extract peptone dextrose (YPD) medium at 30°C (see figure below). A complete cell count with differential was conducted with a result of a total white blood cell (WBC) count of 3,500 cells/mm³, an absolute neutrophil count of 1,700 cells/mm³, and an absolute lymphocyte count of 700 cells/mm³. Flow cytometry detected an absolute CD4 T-cell number of 186 cells/mm³. A fasting glucose level was determined to be 84 mg/dL.

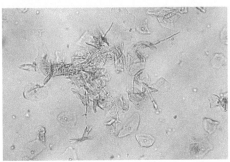

Image courtesy: CDC/ Dr. Stuart Brown

Questions

1. Which of the following is the most likely primary cause of the symptoms which brought her to the doctor?

A. *Candida albicans*

B. *Chlamydia trachomatis*

C. *Gardnerella vaginalis*

D. *Neisseria gonorrhoeae*

E. *Trichomonas vaginalis*

2. Given the patient history and laboratory results what is the most probable underlying reason for the recurrence of these symptoms in this patient?

A. Antibiotic use

B. Diabetes

C. Immunodeficiency

D. Oral contraceptives

E. Sexual transmission

3. Which test is necessary to suggest the cause for the underlying diagnosis?

A. CD4 T-cell count

B. Fasting glucose

C. KOH preparation

D. Vaginal culture

E. Serology

4. Which the following pathogens are most likely the underlying infectious agent based on the patient history and laboratory results?

A. Cytomegalovirus (CMV)

B. Epstein–Barr virus (EBV)

C. Human immunodeficiency virus (HIV)

D. Measles virus

E. Zika virus

5. Which of the following tests would most often be used to confirm the underlying diagnosis?

A. Antigen–antibody test

B. Cell culture

C. DNA test

D. Genotyping test

E. RNA test

Answers and Explanations

1. Correct: *Candida albicans* (A)

Candida albicans is a dimorphic fungus that grows as yeast at 37°C and as hyphal filaments at 30°C. A yeast infection is an overgrowth of *Candida* due to environmental conditions. It is actually not an infection and is not generally considered a sexually transmitted disease. The symptoms of a yeast infection are very similar to other sexually transmitted infections and thus should be diagnosed on both clinical grounds and microbial techniques. Visualization of fungi on wet mount with KOH preparation and in culture is recommended for recurrent episodes of yeast outgrowth and when exposed to fluconazole. Additional culture in selective media such as Chromagar allows for speciation. Vaginal discharge due to *Candida* usually appears as thick and white with the consistency of cottage cheese. However, the color of the discharge is not always a reliable marker. A whiff test that detects a fishy odor to the discharge when exposed to KOH is an indication of a bacterial or parasitic infection unlike the odorless characteristic of *Candida*. Additionally, the vaginal pH is usually in the range of 3.8 to 4.5 and is observed to be less than 4.5 in cases of vulvovaginal candidiasis. A vaginal pH of greater than 4.5 is indicative of a bacterial cause for the symptoms.

B It is an agent of sexually transmitted infections.

C It is an example of a cause of bacterial vaginitis.

D It is an agent of sexually transmitted infections.

E It is an agent of sexually transmitted infections.

2. Correct: Immunodeficiency (C)

Vulvovaginal candidiasis is common in both immunocompetent and immunocompromised women. There are several factors associated with increased occurrence of yeast infections and several are listed as answer choices. The key to the underlying cause in this case is the number of vaginal yeast infections that have occurred with this patient over the past year. Although vaginal yeast infections are not necessarily an indication of immunosuppression alone, the observation of thick white patches on the tongue strongly correlate with immunosuppression.

A The patient does not report any recent antibiotic use.

B Uncontrolled diabetes can impact yeast infections, but this is still due to alterations in the immune system as well as the abundance glucose as a fungal nutrient source. Also as the patient's glucose test is in normal range, this is unlikely.

D This option is incorrect as the patient has denied oral contraceptive use.

E *C. albicans* is not considered to be sexually transmitted.

3. Correct: CD4 T-cell count (A)

Of the laboratory tests ordered, only the CD4 T-cell count would be a more direct test for immunodeficiency. The normal range for the WBC is 4,500 to 11,000 cells/mm³ with 20 to 40% being lymphocytes. The normal CD4 count range is 500 to 1,500 cells/mm³. Lower cell numbers indicate immunodeficiency.

B, C, D, E The glucose test determines a condition of prediabetes or diabetes. KOH preparation is for the detection of *Candida* from other fungal infections. The KOH dissolves any skin cells and debris to allow for easier detection of the fungi. The culture allows for identification of the microbial organisms present depending on the method used. Serology is incorrect because most individuals will have positive serology to *Candida* due to frequent exposure.

4. Correct: Human immunodeficiency virus (HIV) (C)

Options A, C, and D all are viruses that result in immunosuppression. Only HIV infection would result in the CD4 count identified and be associated with both the oral and vulvovaginal candidiasis.

A For CMV immunosuppression is a result of acute infection and is transient.

B EBV is activated from a latency state as a result of immunosuppression.

D For measles virus immunosuppression is a result of acute infection and is transient.
E Zika virus does not cause immunosuppression. It is known for birth defects in pregnant women who are infected.

5. Correct: Antigen–antibody test (A)

According to recent Centers for Disease Control and Prevention (CDC) HIV testing recommendations, initial testing of serum or plasma specimens for HIV should be conducted using Food and Drug Administration (FDA)-approved combination antigen–antibody immunoassay that detects HIV-1, HIV-2, and HIV1 p-24. For reactive samples, confirmatory testing that can differentiate between HIV-1 and HIV-2 antibodies is required.

B HIV is not cultured for routine diagnosis.
C Nonreactive results on the confirmatory testing should be tested with FDA-approved HIV-1 nucleic acid tests.
D Genotyping tests are done for determination of HIV antiretroviral therapy resistance, not diagnosis.
E HIV RNA test is to quantify viral load and is used to determine disease progression, not diagnosis.

Keywords: *Candida*, HIV, resistance, immunodeficiency, diabetes, CMV, measles virus, EBV

Case 28

Adult Male with a Red Eye

A 63-year-old male visits his primary care physician in an urgent basis. The gentleman notes that for the last day, his left eye has been tearing excessively and he feels like there is dirt in his eye. The eye appears red. This morning he noticed pain when looking toward a bright light. Past medical history indicates no previous eye disease. On physical examination, the man had swelling of the eyelid, a red, irritated, tearing left eye and cloudiness of the cornea but was otherwise essentially normal. A fluorescein stain of the cornea of the infected eye under blue light shows microdendritic corneal ulcers with branching lesions and terminal bulbus ends. A scraping of the cornea was sent to the laboratory and was determined negative for Gram stain and growth in culture after 48 hours.

Questions

1. Which of the following pathogens is most likely the cause of the infection in this patient?

A. Adenovirus

B. *Chlamydia trachomatis*

C. Herpes simplex virus (HSV)

D. *Neisseria gonorrhoeae*

E. *Treponema pallidum*

2. What is the most likely cause of transmission of this infection?

A. Airborne transmission

B. Bloodborne transmission

C. Sexual transmission

D. Vertical transmission

E. Waterborne transmission

3. Which of the following laboratory methods would be best considered for diagnosis?

A. Direct fluorescent antibody (DFA)

B. Immunoglobulin M (IgM) titer

C. IgG titer

D. Polymerase chain reaction (PCR)

E. Western blot

4. Besides the ocular infection, which of these presentations is of primary concern for progression of the disease in this individual?

A. Meningoencephalitis

B. Mucositis

C. Osteomyelitis

D. Pneumonia

E. Stromal necrosis

5. Which of the following would be the most appropriate treatment for the patient at this time?

A. Acyclovir, oral

B. Acyclovir, topically

C. Ceftriaxone

D. Erythromycin

E. Vidarabine

Answers and Explanations

1. Correct: Herpes simplex virus (HSV) (C)

This is a case of herpes simplex epithelial keratitis due to HSV infection. Although most infections of this type are caused by bacterial species infections in the United States, all of the answer choices should be considered in the differential. The indication of HSV here is the identification of dendritic lesion on the cornea.

A, B, D, E Adenovirus causes pink eye (conjunctivitis) and is not usually associated with keratitis. *Chlamydia trachomatis* and *Neisseria gonorrhoeae* eye infections occur more often in neonates and are not common in adults. *Treponema pallidum* is not likely because this patient does not have any other apparent symptoms of syphilis; in addition, syphilitic eye infection is more common in neonates and is nonulcerative keratitis.

2. Correct: Sexual transmission (C)

Of the options listed, past sexual transmission is the most likely answer. Ocular herpes virus transmission tends to be HSV-1 instead of HSV-2, however, cases caused by HSV-2 are increasingly being reported.

A, B, D, E HSV is not transmitted via biting insects, airborne, or waterborne routes. While vertical transmission can be a route of transmission for neonatal ophthalmia, this patient is elderly. The most correct answer to describe the scenario is sexual transmission.

3. Correct: Polymerase chain reaction (PCR) (D)

Diagnosis of epithelial keratitis is often based on clinical findings. For diagnostic tests, PCR has become the test of choice in recent years, Although false negatives have been reported. While viral culture was the gold standard for many years, most clinical microbiology laboratories no longer perform viral culture as it requires maintaining cell lines for growing the virus, and

as PCR has become a better test and a test which can be used for many different conditions, it has replaced viral culture.

A, B, C, E Many sources will still list viral culture as the most appropriate test, but its availability has become much more limited. Serology is not always reliable for determining HSV infection as false negatives occur in adults, and serology only confirms exposure and implies past or present infection; it is not a definitive test. DFA is highly specific but can lack sensitivity especially from an area such as the eye where very limited amounts of tissue may be obtained.

4. Correct: Stromal necrosis (E)

The greatest progression risk of this localized ocular HSV manifestation is infection of the stroma. Stromal infection by the virus can lead to an inflammatory response to actively replicating viral particles. This response can result in the destruction of the cornea leading to blindness.

A, B, C, D While all of the listed disease manifestations can be attributed to HSV infection, HSV-1 pneumonia is uncommon and HSV-2 primary infection is more prevalent in HSV meningoencephalitis. Osteomyelitis in HSV-1 infection is not reported.

5. Correct: Acyclovir, oral (A)

For infectious keratitis, debridement of the infected cells using a cotton-tipped applicator prior to any therapy will allow for faster resolution of the condition. Intravenous acyclovir is the treatment of choice for HSV of all types.

B While this appears to be a localized infection, topical therapy is not appropriate as it most likely has spread to the central nervous system (CNS) or disseminated broadly. Intravenous (IV) acyclovir has been shown to reduce progression.

C, D Ceftriaxone is the treatment for *Gonorrhoeae* and erythromycin is the treatment for *Chlamydia.*

E Vidarabine can be used to treat HSV but has significantly higher toxicities than acyclovir.

Keywords: Ophthalmia, sexually transmitted infection, herpetic dendrites, HSV-1

Case 29

Adult Female with Lesion on Labia

A 21-year-old female presented to her gynecologist for routine medical care. She had first been seen by her gynecologist at the age of 16 but had not seen this physician since. She is sexually active and has had five partners since the age of 16. She reports that she uses condoms. She has never been pregnant and has never been diagnosed with a sexually transmitted infection (STI). A pelvic examination was conducted and a single small, flat condyloma was noted on the internal surface of the labia (see figure below). The patient had never noticed it and it is causing no symptoms. An acetowhitening test was done to determine the severity of lesions and noted several areas of blanching of the mucous membranes. A liquid-based Papanicolaou test was done and the cells were sent to the laboratory for evaluation. The pathology report described atypical squamous cells of undetermined significance.

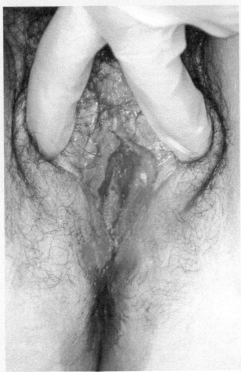

Image courtesy: CDC/ Joe Millar

Questions

1. Which of the following organisms is the most likely causative etiology for these lesions?

A. *Chlamydia trachomatis*

B. Herpes simplex virus

C. Human herpesvirus 6 (HHV-6)

D. Human papillomavirus (HPV)

E. *Treponema pallidum*

2. Which of the following strains is most often associated with genital warts?

A. 6

B. 16

C. 18

D. 33

E. 40

3. This organism has known high- and low-risk strains. For which of the following conditions is this patient at greatest risk of developing, if she is found to be infected with one of these high-risk strains?

A. Breast cancer

B. Cervical cancer

C. Colon cancer

D. Lung cancer

E. Melanoma

4. Which proteins produced by these organisms are associated with oncogenic potential?

A. IncA and IncB

B. gB and gH

C. E6 and E7

D. ICP4 and UL21

E. Tp0155 and Tp0483

5. Which of the following best describes the most appropriate next step in the work-up and treatment considering this patient's abnormal Pap result?

A. Biopsy to confirm the diagnosis of genital warts

B. Cryotherapy to remove the wart and prevent it from spreading to her partners

C. Loop electrosurgical excision procedure (LEEP) to remove all abnormal cells

D. Radical excision of the wart and the areas of blanching in the genital mucosa

E. Repeat examination and Pap smear in 1 year

Answers and Explanations

1. Correct: Human papillomavirus (HPV) (D)

HPV is a DNA virus of the *Papillomaviridae* family. There are over 100 strains of HPV that are identified as sexually and nonsexually transmitted. It is the sexually transmitted viral strains that are the cause of genital warts. HPV is spread by skin-to-skin and mucous membrane contact. The risk factors for infection with sexually transmitted HPV strains are age at first sexual intercourse, having multiple partners, and immune status. The infection can be cleared but risk of viral persistence increases with age of the infected individual.

A, B, C, E The type of lesion described in this case is descriptive of HPV, and not the other sexually transmitted infectious agents listed in the answer choices.

2. Correct: 6 (A)

Strains 6 and 11 account for approximately 90% of genital warts, but are considered low-risk strains for HPV-related cervical and anal cancers.

B, C, D, E Other strains of the virus can cause nongenital warts. Additional low-risk strains are 40, 42, 43, 44, 53, 54, 61, 72, 73, and 81.

3. Correct: Cervical cancer (B)

The high-risk strains 16 and 18 are associated with over 70% of cervical and anal cancers. Additional high-risk strains identified are 31, 33, 35, 39, 45, 51, 52, 56, 58, 59, and 68. There are currently vaccines available that target viral strains 6, 11, 16, and 18, as well as five additional high-risk types. Current recommendations are to vaccinate young men and women beginning at age 11 or 12.

A, C, D, E The high-risk strains are not associated with the other cancer types listed in the answer choices.

4. Correct: E6 and E7 (C)

The viral proteins E6 and E7 are the predominant agents of oncogenic potential from HPV infection. The virus infects keratinocytes and mucosal epithelial cells. The E6 protein interacts with p53 tumor suppressor protein and prevents the infected cell from undergoing apoptosis. Additionally, the E7 protein binds to retinoblastoma tumor suppressor gene product to remove the inhibition on cell growth. Both interactions result in the unchecked growth of infected cells. Abnormal growth of these cells is termed dysplasia and is graded according to progression-relevant staging. Atypical squamous cells of undetermined significance is the lowest grade and triggers continued observation for cancer progression. A level 1 lesion is termed low-grade squamous intraepithelial lesion (LSIL) and is a quantifying term meaning that approximately one-third of cells are abnormal. High-grade squamous intraepithelial lesions (HSILs) are two-thirds abnormal. A severe grading means almost all of the cells are abnormal. For cervical cells these are labeled as cervical intraepithelial neoplasia (CIN) 1, 2, or 3. All are designations for precancerous lesions.

A IncA and IncB are proteins of *Chlamydia trachomatis* involved in regulation of fusion in the endolysosomal pathway relevant to inclusion biogenesis.

B gB and gH are surface glycoproteins that contribute to HHV-6 virus cell fusion.

D ICP4 is a transcriptional regulatory protein and UL21 is a tegument protein of HSV-1.

E Tp0155 and Tp0483 are *Treponema* spp. fibronectin binding proteins. None of these other answer choices are demonstrated to have oncogenic potential.

5. Correct: Repeat examination and Pap smear in 1 year (E)

For women aged 21 to 24, HPV is considered a common finding that will often resolve. Atypical squamous cells of uncertain significance are not an indication that the patient will necessarily develop cervical cancer, and as such they warrant follow-up but not immediate treatment. In this case question, there are two logical choices for follow-up. The first is to send a sample for HPV testing, and if negative, simply resume normal routine testing. The second is to repeat the examination and Pap in 1 year.

A Biopsy is only needed if lesions are atypical (e.g., pigmented, indurated, affixed to underlying tissue, bleeding, or ulcerated lesions). Biopsy also might be indicated in the following circumstances, particularly if the patient is immunocompromised (including those infected with HIV): (1) the diagnosis is uncertain; (2) the lesions do not respond to standard therapy; or (3) the disease worsens during therapy.

Keywords: Genital warts, HPV, cervical cancer

B It has not been shown that cryotherapy reduces infectivity in patients with HPV.

C LEEP is used for removal of precancerous and cancerous cells. As the determination of the Pap was atypical squamous cells of undetermined significance (ASCUS), removal is not warranted at this time.

D Removal of a condyloma (or wart) is generally only for those which are either causing discomfort or are cosmetically unappealing. In this case, the wart was small, flat, and asymptomatic. The patient didn't even know she had it, thus, there is no need for excision or treatment.

Case 30

Adult Male with Back Pain after Trauma

A 35-year-old male presents to the emergency department with back pain from the previous week. He describes the pain as achy on his midback, unrelenting, and limiting of motion. He rates the pain as 7 out of 10. The patient is generally healthy but has had recurrent boils over the last several years that usually spontaneously drain and resolve. He hasn't noted any for the last 4 months. He mentions that he was mugged about a week prior to the pain starting and one of his assailants hit him across the back with a plank of wood. He was assessed by Emergency Medical Services (EMS) at the scene and he appeared to be fine other than some scrapes. When the pain started, he assumed it was bruising from the assault. Physical examination reveals a temperature of 38.8°C. His back is tender to palpation across the spine approximately at the level of T5–T6. There are some scabs and generally well-healed scrapes in the region. Routine bloodwork is drawn and the patient is sent for X-rays. His laboratories show a mild leukocytosis of 12.1 x 10^9 cells/L, a normal complete metabolic profile, an erythrocyte sedimentation rate (ESR) of 85 mm/hr (upper limit of normal 18), and C-reactive protein (CRP) of 9.8 ug/mL (upper limit of normal 0.8). The X-ray comes back showing some subtle soft tissue shadows but normal bone. Given the elevation of the ESR and CRP and the persistent pain, the patient is sent for a magnetic resonance imaging (MRI) of the thoracic spine. The MRI shows a hyperintensity at T5 and T6 which is read as bone marrow edema, as well as loss of endplate definition on the endplates of T5 and T6 and phlegmonous changes, possibly early paraspinal abscess. Blood cultures are drawn and the orthopaedic spine service is called to see the patient. After examination and review of the MRI, they elect to take the patient to surgery where a paraspinal abscess was drained and a bone biopsy was taken. Gram stain of the organism is shown in the figure below. A rapid molecular test indicates the presence of the resistance marker *mecA*. The patient is started on empiric antibiotics.

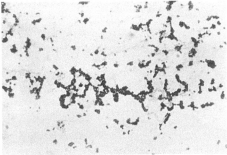

Image courtesy: CDC/ Dr. Richard Facklam

1. Which of the following organisms is the most likely causative agent?

A. *Clostridium perfringens*

B. *Pseudomonas aeruginosa*

C. *Salmonella enterica*

D. *Staphylococcus aureus*

E. *Streptococcus pyogenes*

2. Which of the following laboratory test results would you expect for the most likely causative agent?

Options	Catalase	Coagulase	Oxacillin
A.	+	+	Sensitive
B.	−	+	Sensitive
C.	−	−	Sensitive
D.	+	+	Resistant
E.	−	+	Resistant

A. Option A

B. Option B

C. Option C

D. Option D

E. Option E

3. Which of the following virulence factors would be most likely produced from this organism?

A. Edema factor

B. M protein

C. Panton–Valentine leukocidin (PVL) toxin

D. Tetanospasmin

E. Toxic shock syndrome toxin-1 (TSST-1)

4. Which of the following describes the most likely source of this pathogen in this infection?

A. Hematogenous spread

B. Arthropod bite

C. Contact with an infected person

D. Water contamination

E. Direct inoculation

5. Given what is known about the patient's infection and the likely organism that caused it, which of the following antibioGrams is most likely to be found when sensitivities result?

A. Penicillin−S, methicillin−S, clindamycin−S, bactrim−S, vancomycin−S

B. Penicillin−R, methicillin−S, clindamycin−S, bactrim−S, vancomycin−S

C. Penicillin−R, methicillin−R, clindamycin−S, bactrim−S, vancomycin−S

D. Penicillin−R, methicillin−R, clindamycin−R, bactrim−R, vancomycin−S

E. Penicillin−R, methicillin−R, clindamycin−R, bactrim−R, vancomycin−R

1. Correct: *Staphylococcus aureus* (D)

The patient's symptoms, imaging, and laboratory findings describe vertebral osteomyelitis. In adults, the most common route of infection for vertebral osteomyelitis is hematogenous and the infections are typically monomicrobial with *Staphylococcus aureus* being the most common causative agent. This patient, however, describes a history of boils which is also typically caused by *S. aureus*. This is generally resulting from community-acquired methicillin-resistant *S. aureus* (CA-MRSA). Most patients who have recurrent episodes of boils are colonized with CA-MRSA on their skin, and the direct injury sustained when the patient was mugged gives a likely cause for the deeper infection. The Gram stain shown in the figure supports this finding as gram-positive cocci can be seen arranged in typical cluster patterns. Other causes of vertebral osteomyelitis are coagulase-negative *Staphylococcus*, aerobic gram-negative bacilli, *Streptococcus* spp., *Enterococcus* spp., anaerobes, fungi, and *Mycobacterium* spp.

A *Clostridium perfringens* are gram-positive bacilli.

B, C *Pseudomonas aeruginosa* and *S. enterica* are gram-negative bacilli.

E While *Streptococcus pyogenes* are gram-positive cocci, they are not common causative agents of osteomyelitis, and so *S. aureus* is the best answer.

2. Correct: Option D (D)

This patient has osteomyelitis caused by *S. aureus*. *S. aureus* are gram-positive cocci that are catalase positive and coagulase positive. The case presentation reveals that the causative agent was likely CA-MRSA given the history of boils and detection of *mecA*, which is the gene that codes for resistance to nafcillin, oxacillin, and methicillin.

A This describes methicillin-sensitive *S. aureus* (MSSA).

B Catalase negative bacteria include *Streptococcus* and *Enterococcus* Coagulase activity is a test that distinguishes *S. Aureus* (+) from other *Staphylococcus* species.

C Catalase negative bacteria include *Streptococcus* and *Enterococcus*, which are also coagulase negative. Coagulase negative *Staphylococcus* species would not be catalase negative.

E This describes methicillin-resistant *S. aureus* MRSA.

3. Correct: Panton–Valentine leukocidin (PVL) toxin (C)

This case describes a patient with osteomyelitis caused by a strain of CA-MRSA. CA-MRSA strains carry a large genetic island called the staphylococcal cassette chromosome which codes for its resistance gene (*mecA*) and also often codes for various virulence factors. Most strains of CA-MRSA produce PVL, believed to play a role in the pathogenesis of the infection.

A Edema factor is a toxin produced by *Bacillus anthracis*.

B M protein is produced by *S. pyogenes*, and certain strains are associated with rheumatic fever.

D Tetanospasmin is a toxin produced by *Clostridium tetani*.

E TSST-1 toxin is produced by some strains of *S. aureus*. Although some MRSA strains will produce TSST-1, the MRSA strain that is causing the infection described here would not be expected to produce TSST-1 during an osteomyelitis infection.

4. Correct: Direct inoculation (E)

MRSA is transmitted by contact from patient to patient or from surfaces or fomites to patients, but this generally causes colonization and not an immediate infection. When a patient is colonized by the pathogen, it makes up a portion of the normal flora of the individual. At times, the colonizing bacteria can cause an actual infection when those bacteria reach a normally sterile site. This case describes osteomyelitis where transmission was likely endogenous from the patient's own normal skin flora, and likely entered via direct inoculation when the patient was mugged and struck across the back by a plank, causing scrapes and likely splinters.

A Hematogenous spread is via the blood stream. This type of transmission was less likely in this case.

B *S. aureus* is not normally transmitted through arthropod bites.

C As described previously, person to person spread is not likely given the scenario of this case.

D *S. aureus* is not a waterborne pathogen.

5. Correct: Penicillin—R, methicillin—R, clindamycin—S, bactrim—S, vancomycin—S (C)

This question asks for a determination of the sensitivity pattern of the organism based solely on limited information. We know the causative agent is a strain of MRSA, due to the presence of the mecA gene, and that it is likely CA-MRSA.

A This option is incorrect because most strains of *S. aureus* are resistant to penicillin.

B MRSA are resistant to nafcillin, oxacillin, and methicillin (the three anti-staphylococcal penicillins). Almost all MRSA strains are sensitive to vancomycin. Vancomycin-resistant *S. aureus* (VRSA) is extremely rare with only 13 cases reported in the United States to date.

D, E These options are incorrect as most strains of MRSA remain sensitive to bactrim and it is frequently used to treat simple MRSA infections, such as those found in the skin and soft tissue. Most strains of CA-MRSA remain sensitive to clindamycin, which is often considered a good choice for treatment of CAMRSA infections since it is a protein synthesis inhibitor that can have the secondary function of shutting down production of toxins and other virulence factors often found in CA-MRSA.

Keywords: *Staphylococcus aureus*, MRSA, osteomyelitis, vancomycin, catalase, coagulase

Case 31

Teenage Girl with Expanding Skin Lesion

A 15-year-old adolescent girl presents with her parents to her family physician with skin lesions that appeared while recovering from a varicella infection. Past medical history indicates that the patient is diabetic and has only completed some portions of the required vaccinations. The patient has not been previously vaccinated for varicella. Her mother tells the physician that the patient works part-time at a pet store. Both parents are employed by the military and the family moves frequently. She states that the lesions have been present for approximately 1 day and that she first noticed her varicella rash 6 days previously. Physical examination reveals numerous healing crusted over vesicular lesions and on the left arm there is an erythematous area with a violaceous dusky center. The main area that started as a small red patch is now about 5 cm in diameter and has extended up the arm toward the shoulder and the elbow. The area is exquisitely tender and even mild pressure causes the girl to cry out in pain. Enlarged axillary lymph nodes are also noted. Her temperature is 38.9°C and her blood pressure (BP) is 95/55 mmHg. Emergency Medical Services (EMS) is called and the patient is rapidly transferred to the emergency department at the local hospital. During the 20-minute drive, her mother notices that the lesions seem to look more serious and have progressed even further, now extending past the elbow with increased duskiness. Upon arrival at the emergency department, the patient is rapidly examined by multiple physicians, has antibiotics started, and is rushed to surgery. Blood is drawn for aerobic and anaerobic cultures and material from the lesion is obtained during surgery and sent for culture. Both sources are found to contain a single organism, which is shown on the Gram stain in the figure below.

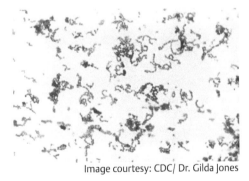

Image courtesy: CDC/ Dr. Gilda Jones

Questions

1. Which of the following organisms is the most likely causative agent?

A. *Enterobacter cloacae*

B. *Enterococcus faecalis*

C. *Staphylococcus aureus*

D. *Streptococcus pneumoniae*

E. *Streptococcus pyogenes*

2. For the most likely causative agent, which of the following is a major virulence factor related to this condition?

A. Lipopolysaccharide (LPS)

B. M protein

C. Exotoxin A

D. Protein A

E. Immunoglobulin A (IgA) protease

3. Which of the following best describes the hemolysis expected from the most likely causative agent?

A. α (alpha) hemolysis

B. β (beta) hemolysis

C. δ (delta) hemolysis

D. ε (epsilon) hemolysis

E. γ (gamma) hemolysis

4. Which of the following is a risk factor for this patient for the development of necrotizing fasciitis?

A. Age

B. Diabetes

C. Exposure to pets

D. Incomplete vaccination history

E. Residing with an active member of the military

5. What is the most appropriate therapy for this patient after receiving the Gram stain result?

A. Vancomycin

B. Ampicillin/Sulbactam

C. Vancomycin + piperacillin/tazobactam + clindamycin

D. Penicillin + clindamycin

E. Penicillin + Gentamicin

Answers and Explanations

1. Correct: *Streptococcus pyogenes* (E)

This patient has necrotizing fasciitis. Without immediate intervention, these infections have a high mortality rate. Diabetes is a risk factor, as well as the fact that this patient had a recent skin infection (with the virus varicella zoster). Necrotizing fasciitis can be either polymicrobial or due to *Streptococcus pyogenes* (also known as Group A streptococci [GAS]). The Gram stain in the figure shows gram-positive (purple) cocci in chains, thereby indicating that the causative agent is *S. pyogenes*. With the exception of *Enterobacter cloacae* (which is a gram-negative bacilli, and therefore not the correct answer based on the Gram stain alone), all of the other choices listed are gram-positive cocci, so the arrangement of the cocci on the Gram stain is important.

A, B, C, D *Staphylococcus aureus* are cocci arranged as clusters on a Gram stain, whereas the Gram stain associated with this case indicates an arrangement of the cocci in chains. The remaining choices *Enterococcus faecalis, Streptococcus pneumoniae,* and *S. pyogenes* are gram-positive cocci that are often arranged in chains or pairs, and so all three are feasible answers based on the Gram stain alone. However, only *S. pyogenes* is associated with the clinical signs of necrotizing fasciitis that are described in the case. Furthermore, *S. pneumoniae* is often arranged in pairs or short chains on Gram stain, not the longer chains that are seen in the figure.

2. Correct: M protein (B)

This case describes a patient with necrotizing fasciitis due to *S. pyogenes*. A major virulence determinant of *S. pyogenes* is the M protein. The M protein is located on the bacterial cell surface and aids in the prevention of phagocytosis by macrophages, thereby allowing for further bacterial growth during infection. The type 1 and type 3 M protein are most often associated with necrotizing fasciitis, while other types are associated with rheumatic fever. In addition, pyrogenic exotoxins A, B, or C are often produced by bacterial strains associated with necrotizing fasciitis (though those exotoxins are not a choice in this question).

A *S. pyogenes* is a gram-positive organism, and only gram-negative bacteria produce LPS.

C *S. pyogenes* do not produce exotoxin A (a toxin produced by *Pseudomonas aeruginosa*).

D Protein A is a virulence factor of *S. aureus*, not *S. pyogenes*.

E IgA protease is a virulence factor produced by some strains of *S. pneumoniae*, *Haemophilus influenzae* type B, and *Neisseria* spp. that aids in the colonization of the respiratory mucosa. *S. pyogenes* do not produce IgA protease.

3. Correct: β (beta) hemolysis (B)

This case describes necrotizing fasciitis caused by *S. pyogenes*. *S. pyogenes* is also known as GAS or group A beta-hemolytic *Streptococcus* (GABHS). When grown on agar plates containing blood, bacterial colonies are surrounded by zones of complete clearing, due to total hemolysis of the red blood cells in the media. Complete hemolysis is termed beta hemolysis.

A Partial hemolysis of the red blood cells is termed alpha hemolysis, and often leads to a greenish color zone surrounding each bacterial colony.

C, D The terms delta and epsilon hemolysis do not exist.

E The term that describes no hemolysis of red blood cells is gamma hemolysis.

4. Correct: Diabetes (B)

Diabetes is a risk factor for the development of necrotizing fasciitis. Other important risk factors include drug use, obesity, immunosuppression (including prolonged corticosteroid therapy), recent surgery, malnutrition, and traumatic wounds.

A Advanced age is also a risk factor, but in this case, the patient is 15 years old, so that is not a risk factor.

C Exposure to pets from the patient's place of employment would possibly make her more at risk for zoonotic infections such as cat scratch disease (*Bartonella henselae*), *Leptospira* spp., *Salmonella* spp., or rabies virus.

D There is no vaccine for *S. pyogenes*, so vaccination would not protect this patient from the infection.

E There is no mention of military service in the case.

5. Correct: Penicillin + clindamycin (D)

Surgical debridement is the cornerstone of treatment of necrotizing fasciitis. All the antibiotics in the world will not cure the patient if dead tissue is not removed. Empiric antibiotic treatment for necrotizing fasciitis must include broad-spectrum antibiotics to cover a mixed infection and the possibility of methicillin-resistant *S. aureus* (MRSA) and should include a protein synthesis inhibitor such as clindamycin for toxin inhibition. However, once it is clear that the infection is due to GAS, the treatment can be narrowed and penicillin plus clindamycin is the preferred regimen. An aminoglycoside such as gentamicin (and vancomycin) also inhibits protein synthesis but has much more significant dosing challenges and side effects than clindamycin, as well as less inherent activity against gram-positive organisms.

A Vancomycin is inappropriate because *S. pyogenes* does not need to be treated with vancomycin and in this clinical scenario, the addition of a protein synthesis inhibitor such as clindamycin is required.

B Ampicillin–sulbactam would be indicated but is overly broad, and would also require the addition of a protein synthesis inhibitor.

C Vancomycin + piperacillin–tazobactam + clindamycin is overly broad.

E While gentamicin is a protein synthesis inhibitor, its activity is primarily against gram-negatives and its toxicities (primarily nephrotoxicity) should be avoided when there is a reasonable alternative such as clindamycin.

Keywords: Necrotizing fasciitis, *Streptococcus pyogenes*, Group A *Streptococcus*, M protein, beta-hemolysis

Case 32

Adult Male with Foot Ulcer

A 45-year-old male presents to a free clinic with an ulcer on the sole of his left foot at the base of the toes, with exposed bone. The toes are cold and clearly losing the skin, and there are black lesions over the toes where the skin is lost. There is a malodorous smell which is easily noted. The patient says that he first noticed the discoloration 2 days earlier and that it is painful even though his feet are usually numb. The man is currently homeless and has been living in the outdoors around a large city for the previous 4 months. He says that his only pair of shoes is too small, so he tends to walk barefoot whenever possible. He also says that he finds that he stumbles frequently.

The patient doesn't provide much medical history; however, he states that he was previously told that he was "mildly diabetic" and the doctors wanted to start him on medications, but he could not afford the medication, so he has never been treated. He denies ever having issues like this before but does note that his feet tend to have numbness. He also sometimes experiences shooting pains which he describes as "electric" for more than a year. He also recalls being in the hospital about 10 years earlier to have his appendix removed.

The patient states that he has a girlfriend but that she does not have similar symptoms. He doesn't know anything about his family history and he denies alcohol or recreational drug use.

Physical examination reveals a temperature of 38.2°C, blood pressure of 95/60 mmHg, and heart rate of 120 bpm. The left foot displays edema and a thin, dark, malodorous discharge from the ulcer on the sole. Crepitus is present, but he does not react to pressure on the area. A bedside fingerstick reveals a blood sugar of 280. An X-ray of the foot shows a soft tissue defect consistent with the ulcer, generalized edema in the area, periosteal reaction in the bones of the foot and toes and gas throughout the forefoot, and tracking toward the heel.

Bloodwork including cultures are drawn and a deep swab from the wound is collected and sent for Gram stain, aerobic and anaerobic cultures. The Gram stain from the wound is shown in the figure below. Cultures grew multiple organisms, the most prominent were gram-positive cocci in clusters, gram-positive bacilli that are obligate anaerobes and grow with a double zone of hemolysis on blood agar, and aerobic gram-negative bacilli.

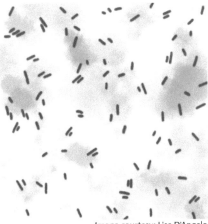

Image courtesy: Lisa D'Angelo

Questions

1. Which of the following organisms is the most likely causative agent of the gas noted on the X-ray and the crepitus?

A. *Bacillus anthracis*

B. *Clostridium perfringens*

C. *Pasteurella multocida*

D. *Pseudomonas aeruginosa*

E. *Staphylococcus saprophyticus*

2. Which of the following bacterial characteristics would most likely confirm your suspicion of the identity of the gram-positive anaerobic organism?

A. Ability to form spores

B. Acid-fast stain red

C. Catalase positive

D. Growth at 25°C in a standard incubator

E. Oxidase positive

3. For the most likely gram-positive anaerobe, which of the following best describes a toxin that is produced during the infection?

A. Alpha toxin

B. Edema factor

C. Exotoxin A

D. Lipopolysaccharide (LPS)

E. Tetanospasmin

4. Which of the following is the most likely source of the gram-positive anaerobe?

A. Endogenous

B. Previous surgery

C. Respiratory droplets

D. Sexual transmission

E. Soil

5. At this point, which of the following would be the most appropriate therapy to cure this infection?

A. Broad-spectrum antibiotics including coverage for gram-positives, *Pseudomonas*, and anaerobes

B. Narrow-spectrum antibiotics focusing on anaerobes and with a protein synthesis inhibitor for its antitoxin properties

C. Broad-spectrum antibiotics plus debridement of necrotic tissue

D. Broad-spectrum antibiotics plus a below-the-knee amputation

E. Broad-spectrum antibiotics plus hyperbaric oxygen therapy

Answers and Explanations

1. Correct: *Clostridium perfringens* (B)

This case describes a soft tissue polymicrobial infection. These types of mixed infections are usually caused by both anaerobic and aerobic organisms, as can be seen in the Gram stain of the wound exudate. The Gram stain shows both gram-positive and gram-negative bacilli. Diabetes is a risk factor due to the decrease in vascular supply, especially in the extremities. Organisms are usually introduced into subcutaneous tissue via trauma, in this case likely a foot puncture from walking barefoot in the outdoors. Pain despite typical neuropathy and numbness of the feet, swelling, gas on the X-ray, and crepitus are often seen in clostridial infections, caused by *Clostridium perfringens*. *C. perfringens* are gram-positive bacilli that are spore-forming, obligate anaerobes. The bacteria characteristically grow with a double zone of hemolysis on blood agar, as described in this case.

A *Bacillus anthracis* do clinically manifest as a black eschar, and are gram-positive bacilli; however, they are facultative anaerobes and do not grow with a double zone of hemolysis. Infections with *B. anthracis* also do not commonly cause crepitus; they are also extremely rare in the United States and generally are caused from exposure to animal fur.

C *Pasteurella multocida* is involved with dog-bite infections, and there was no mention of an animal bite in this case. Furthermore, *P. multocida* are facultative anaerobes and infections do not often cause crepitus or a black lesion.

D *Pseudomonas aeruginosa* are commonly seen in diabetic foot infections but are not typically gas producers and do not generally cause crepitus.

E *Staphylococcus saprophyticus* is involved with urinary tract infections and are gram-positive cocci.

2. Correct: Ability to form spores (A)

The gram-positive organism in this case is likely *C. perfringens*, causing the gangrene that is described in this patient. *C. perfringens* are spore-forming gram-positive bacilli that are obligate anaerobes. These organisms will form endospores under harsh conditions in the environment to enhance survival.

B *C. perfringens* are non–acid-fast organisms and would therefore stain blue with an acid-fast stain.

C, D, E A catalase or oxidase test would not be used to identify *C. perfringens*, but the organisms are catalase negative and oxidase negative as well. These organisms are obligate anaerobes, so while they would grow at 25°C, they would not be able to survive the oxygen conditions of a standard incubator.

3. Correct: Alpha toxin (A)

The most likely gram-positive causative agent in this case is *C. perfringens*. During soft tissue infections, these bacteria produce many exotoxins, including alpha and theta toxins. Alpha toxin is a hemolytic toxin that has phospholipase C (PLC) and sphingomyelinase activities. Alpha toxin is essential for pathogenesis of *C. perfringens*, and the toxin degrades host tissues and cell membranes, leading to gangrene and other soft tissue infections.

B Edema factor is an exotoxin produced by *B anthracis*; however *B anthracis* is not the causative agent in the case (see Question 1).

C Exotoxin A is an exotoxin produced by *P. aeruginosa*, a gram-negative facultative anaerobe. The enzymatic activity of exotoxin A results in host cell death by ADP-ribosylating elongation factor 2 (EF-2) and halting protein synthesis in host cells.

D LPS is the endotoxin present in nearly all gram-negative bacteria (*C. perfringens* is gram-positive and therefore does not produce LPS).

E Tetanospasmin is an exotoxin produced by *Clostridium tetani*, the causative agent of tetanus and lockjaw.

4. Correct: Soil (E)

This case describes a soft tissue infection caused by *C. perfringens*. These bacteria are found in the environment in the soil and also in marine sediments. They are also found in the intestinal tract of humans and animals. Human infections result following trauma, which introduces the organisms directly into the tissues. Both the vegetative and spore forms of the organism may be introduced into the body prior to infection. These organisms require anaerobic conditions for growth, so any condition that has a compromised vascular supply (such as diabetes) will enhance growth of these organisms.

A While *C. perfringens* are often inhabitants of the human gastrointestinal tract, infections are rarely endogenous and the organisms are nearly always acquired from the environment (soil).

B This patient mentions a previous surgery; however, it would be extremely unlikely that the surgical wound would be contaminated with *C. perfringens* if normal sterile conditions were present. Furthermore, the surgery was a decade earlier, and most bacterial infections do not have such a long incubation period.

C, D *C. perfringens* are not transmitted via respiratory droplets or sexual transmission.

5. Correct: Broad-spectrum antibiotics plus a below-the-knee amputation (D)

This is a case of serious, life-threatening gangrene of the foot as evidenced by gas throughout the foot, rapid development, systemic symptoms, evidence of osteomyelitis, and loss of circulation. The most appropriate therapy is radical resection in this case with a below-the-knee amputation. If it were more localized, an attempt to save part of the foot with a transmetatarsal amputation could be attempted but that is unlikely to be a viable strategy here given the extent of the infection. Given the systemic symptoms it would be appropriate to have the patient on broad-spectrum antibiotics at least until the amputation is finished, blood cultures are negative, and the patient stabilizes.

A, B, C, E Since source control will be achieved with an amputation that clearly removes the entire infection, the patient will not need a long course of antibiotics to treat osteomyelitis. Antibiotics, whether broad or narrow, alone will not be sufficient to cure this infection. While hyperbaric oxygen may have some role in nonhealing ulcers and anaerobic infections, it is not life-saving in the case of diffuse gangrene.

Keywords: Gangrene, *Clostridium perfringenes*, alpha toxin, diabetes, soft tissue

Case 33

Adult Male with Flu-Like Illness and Rash

A 53-year-old male presents to his primary care physician in August with flu-like symptoms. He complains of a headache, joint pain, mild fever, fatigue, and chills for the past 4 days. He just returned the week before from a week-long family trip to Pennsylvania where he and his family were fishing and hiking. but no one else in the family is sick. His physical examination reveals a temperature of 38°C and mild tachycardia with a heart rate of 103. His physical examination is fairly normal with some tenderness noted at the wrists and shoulders. When he removes his shirt, a rash (shown in the first figure below) can be seen across the back of the patient's right shoulder. Bloodwork is drawn for an enzyme-linked immunosorbent assay (ELISA) test and confirmatory Western blot tests for the suspected causative agent. A skin biopsy revealed the organisms by direct fluorescent antibody (DFA) as shown in the second figure.

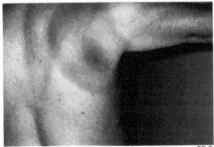

Image courtesy: CDC

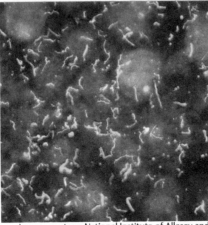

Image courtesy: National Institute of Allergy and Infectious Diseases (NIAID)

Questions

1. Which of the following organisms is the most likely causative agent?

A. *Bartonella henselae*

B. *Borrelia burgdorferi*

C. *Ehrlichia ewingii*

D. *Leptospira interrogans*

E. *Rickettsia rickettsii*

2. What is the vector that most often transmits this infection to humans?

A. *Anopheles* spp.

B. Armadillo

C. *Dermacentor* spp.

D. *Ixodes* spp.

E. Mouse

3. Which of the following is an important virulence factor of the most likely causative agent?

A. Endotoxin

B. Exotoxin

C. Flagella

D. Immunoglobulin A (IgA) protease

E. Pili

4. Which of the following best describes the oxygen metabolism of the most likely causative agent?

A. Aerotolerant anaerobe

B. Facultative

C. Microaerophile

D. Obligate aerobe

E. Obligate anaerobe

5. At this point in his disease which of the following is the most appropriate treatment?

A. Doxycycline 100 mg by mouth twice a day for 14 days

B. Ceftriaxone 2 g IV q12 hours

C. Metronidazole 500 mg by mouth q8 hours

D. Trimethoprim–sulfamethoxazole DS, one tab by mouth q12 hours

E. Ciprofloxacin 400 mg IV q12 hours

Answers and Explanations

Midwestern United States. Clinical features are similar to Lyme disease and so *Rickettsia* should be in the differential diagnosis.

1. Correct: *Borrelia burgdorferi* (B)

This patient has Lyme disease, caused by *Borrelia burgdorferi*. The classical bull's eye rash (erythema migrans) is described on the patient's back. He also describes a history of being in the outdoors in the geographic area of the United States where Lyme disease is endemic, and during the time of year that the vector (ticks) is typically seen. In most cases when the rash is seen, it is a single rash. However, it is estimated that in approximately 10 to 18% of cases multiple erythema migrans rashes may not be visible. The peak ages of those infected are ages 5 to 14 and 50 to 59. *B. burgdorferi* is a spirochete and can be seen in a DFA. It can be visualized with immunofluorescence (as shown here), or with a silver stain from skin biopsies.

A *Bartonella henselae* is the causative agent of cat scratch disease and are small gram-negative bacilli, not spirochetes.

C *Ehrlichia ewingii* cause human granulocytic ehrlichiosis (HGE). *E. ewingii* can also be transmitted by ticks; however, they are small gram-negative rods that are obligately intracellular and are not normally associated with a rash.

D *Leptospira interrogans* is the causative agent of leptospirosis. They are spirochetes and would look similar to the organisms seen in the figure; however, infection of humans is most commonly associated with exposure to infected animal urine or tissue (not mentioned in this case). Furthermore, leptospirosis is more common in the tropics and is associated with risk factors such as poverty and occupational exposure (not mentioned in this case).

E *Rickettsia rickettsii* is the causative agent of Rocky Mountain spotted fever (RMSF). *R. rickettsii* are obligate intracellular gram-negative bacilli (not spirochetes as are seen in the figure). While they are also transmitted by ticks, the geographic distribution includes the South Atlantic and

2. Correct: *Ixodes* spp. (D)

The vector most commonly associated with transmission of *B. burgdorferi* is the *Ixodes* spp. tick. The most common species implicated in transmission are *Ixodes ricinus*, *Ixodes scapularis*, *Ixodes pacificus*, and *Ixodes persulcatus*. Other tick species may harbor the bacteria but are unable to transmit the infection.

A The *Anopheles* spp. is the mosquito vector for *Plasmodium malariae*, *Plasmodium vivax*, *Plasmodium ovale*, and *Plasmodium falciparum*, the causative agents of malaria.

B Armadillos are the reservoir for *Mycobacterium leprae*, and eating these animals is associated with transmission.

C *Dermacentor* spp. are the tick vector associated with *R. rickettsii*, the causative agent to RMSF.

E The mouse is the reservoir for *B. burgdorferi*, not the vector. Other small mammals have also been implicated as reservoirs for *B. burgdorferi*, but there is no evidence that deer may act as a reservoir.

3. Correct: Flagella (C)

B. burgdorferi are motile spirochetes that express flagella for motility. The flagella are located between the inner and outer membranes and facilitate the characteristic corkscrew motility.

A *Borrelia* spp. do not produce lipid A and therefore do not produce endotoxin. However, lipoproteins are present on the surface that act as toll-like receptors.

B These bacteria do not produce exotoxins or proteases during infection, and infection is due primarily to migrating through tissues, colonizing host cell surfaces, and disseminating into the bloodstream.

D Furthermore, the bacteria enter the body via an arthropod bite, so initial infection is not at a mucosal surface (IgA protease would be useless).

E *B. burgdorferi* has not been reported to express pili or fimbriae.

4. Correct: Microaerophile (C)

B. burgdorferi are microaerophilic organisms that require oxygen but grow optimally under conditions of reduced oxygen (5-10%). These are the conditions typical of the small mammal reservoir where these bacteria are normally found. These organisms are fastidious when grown in vitro as they are unable to survive high temperatures, drying, disinfectants, and they require specialized media for growth such as Barbour-Stoenner-Kelly (BSK) media.

A, B, D, E *B. burgdorferi* is unable to survive in obligate aerobic or facultative conditions. Likewise, the organisms are not aerotolerant because they are unable to survive in high oxygen atmospheric conditions. Interestingly, *B. burgdorferi* are able to grow slowly under obligate anaerobic conditions; however, microaerophilic conditions are optimal for growth, therefore they are classified as microaerophiles.

5. Correct: Doxycycline 100 mg by mouth twice a day for 14 days (A)

While there is a great deal of controversy over the diagnosis and treatment of Lyme disease, the current evidence-based guidelines suggest treatment for early Lyme disease, which is what the description of this patient indicates. The treatment should be oral and the first-line treatments include amoxicillin, doxycycline, and cefuroxime. Of these doxycycline is the only choice listed as an answer.

B, C, D, E Ceftriaxone is useful when parenteral treatment is needed, though the dose listed here is a meningitic dose, whereas the dose recommended by the guidelines is the standard 2 g IV daily.

Guidelines indicate: "Because of a lack of biologic plausibility, lack of efficacy, absence of supporting data, or the potential for harm to the patient, the following are not recommended for treatment of patients with any manifestation of Lyme disease: first-generation cephalosporins, fluoroquinolones, carbapenems, vancomycin, metronidazole, tinidazole, amantadine, ketolides, isoniazid, trimethoprim–sulfamethoxazole, fluconazole, benzathine penicillin G, combinations of antimicrobials, pulsed-dosing (i.e., dosing on some days but not others), long-term antibiotic therapy, anti-*Bartonella* therapies, hyperbaric oxygen, ozone, fever therapy, intravenous immunoglobulin, cholestyramine, intravenous hydrogen peroxide, specific nutritional supplements, and others." The remaining choices are all listed in this section of the guidelines.

Keywords: Lyme disease, *Borrelia burgdorferi*, erythema migrans, *Ixodes* spp., tick, spirochete, doxycycline

Case 34

Febrile Teenager with Disseminated Rash

A 13-year old adolescent boy is brought to the pediatrician by his father in June. The family lives in the suburbs of Raleigh, North Carolina, on the edge of a wooded area with their pets, including a cat and two dogs. For the past 3 days the patient has had a fever as high as 103°F, belly pain, and muscle aches. He is listless and doesn't want to eat. Yesterday, he developed a rash that the father says first started on the boy's feet and hands and then moved to his trunk and face (see figure below). The lesions are small macules, are not pruritic, and are also found on the palms and soles. The patient's father said he knew he was very sick when he showed no interest in going outside to play with his friends. The patient normally spends at least 2 hours playing in the woods every day, especially since school ended for the summer.

Past medical history indicates that the patient has only completed a portion of the required immunizations. Vital signs include a temperature of 104.5°F, pulse 155, and blood pressure 105/65 mmHg. Other than the rash, the notable findings on the examination included conjunctival injection, abdominal tenderness, and lethargy. Blood is drawn for routine laboratory examination and white blood cell count is normal, but the patient is thrombocytopenic with a platelet count of 145. His liver function tests are above the upper limit of normal but less than 2× above the upper limit. A skin biopsy with direct immunofluorescence staining reveals intracellular gram-negative coccobacilli.

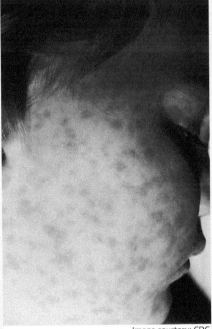

Image courtesy: CDC

Questions

1. Which of the following organisms is the most likely causative agent?

A. *Anaplasma phagocytophilum*

B. *Borrelia burgdorferi*

C. *Leptospira interrogans*

D. *Rickettsia rickettsii*

E. *Yersinia pestis*

2. Which of the following is the vector that transmits this infection to humans?

A. *Sarcoptes scabiei*

B. *Culex pipiens*

C. *Dermacentor variabilis*

D. *Phthirus pubis*

E. *Ixodes scapularis*

3. Which of the following is the best prevention for this infection?

A. Active vaccination

B. Apply repellent containing 20% DEET

C. Avoid pets

D. Avoid mouse droppings

E. Passive vaccination

4. Inside which of the following eukaryotic subcellular locations is the causative agent able to grow and proliferate?

A. Endoplasmic reticulum

B. Golgi apparatus

C. Lysosome

D. Mitochondria

E. Nucleus

5. Given the patient's symptoms and age what is the most appropriate treatment for this infection?

A. Doxycycline

B. Levofloxacin

C. Meropenem

D. Penicillin G

E. Trimethoprim–sulfamethoxazole

Answers and Explanations

This case describes Rocky Mountain spotted fever (RMSF), which is caused by the bacteria *Rickettsia rickettsii*. RMSF is a tick-borne infection that is seen in the United States, Canada, Mexico, Central America, and South America. In the United States, it is most prevalent in the southeastern and south-central states, such as North Carolina. Individuals who are exposed to ticks in the spring and early summer (such as the child in this case who enjoys playing in the woods in June) are most susceptible to infection. Classic clinical manifestations include a fever, headache, muscle aches, and rash. In children, the headache is sometimes missing and they are frequently listless with abdominal pain and conjunctival injection. There are two types of rash associated with RMSF. The early rash is characteristically on the palms of the hands and the soles of the feet and spreads from the ankles and wrists to the trunk; it is macular and nonpruritic. It generally appears between 2 and 5 days, earlier in children and later in adults. Ninety percent of patients develop the rash, but given the potential mortality of RMSF a high clinical suspicion in the right circumstances must be maintained and treatment started. The later rash is petechial and usually does not appear before the sixth day and only occurs in 35 to 60% of patients with RMSF. The appearance of the petechial rash indicates progression to a more severe presentation of the disease, and it is imperative to start treatment before the petechial rash appears. The causative agents of RMSF, *R. rickettsii*, are intracellular gram-negative coccobacilli.

A, B, C, E The other answer choices are incorrect. *Borrelia burgdorferi* is the causative agent of Lyme disease and does not manifest as a diffuse rash, but instead as a "bull's eye rash" also known as erythema migrans. Furthermore, *B. burgdorferi* is a gram-negative spirochete that is rarely, if ever, intracellular during infection.

Leptospira interrogans are gram-negative spirochetes that cause Leptospirosis. Infection is often associated with exposure to infected rodents and rarely manifests as a rash. *Yersinia pestis* is the causative agent of plague. These bacteria are gram-negative coccobacilli with bipolar staining but are usually extracellular. Clinical manifestations rarely include a rash. Both rodents and fleas are involved with transmission of *Y. pestis*. *Anaplasma phagocytophilum* is the causative agent of anaplasmosis which was formerly called ehrlichiosis. It is carried by the *Ixodes* tick much like *Borrelia burgdorferi*. The symptoms of anaplasmosis are similar to RMSF and the treatment is the same but the presence of a rash is rare. Anaplasmosis is sometimes called spotless RMSF.

Dermacentor spp. are the tick vector associated with *R. rickettsii*, the causative agent of the infection described in this case, RMSF. The species varies throughout the country: in the eastern and south central United States, it is *Dermacentor variabilis* (American dog tick); in the mountain states west of the Mississippi River, it is *Dermacentor andersoni* (Rocky Mountain wood tick), and in the southeastern United States, it is a different tick species: *Rhipicephalus sanguineus* (common brown dog tick).

A, B, D, E *Culex* spp. is the primary mosquito vector for West Nile virus. The vector most commonly associated with transmission of *B. burgdorferi*, the causative agent of Lyme disease, as well as *A. phagocytophilum* is the *Ixodes* spp. tick. *Sarcoptes scabiei* are the cause of scabies and *P. pubis* are pubic lice.

This case describes RMSF, and prevention is primarily by avoidance of the tick vector. Prevention of tick bites can be by wearing proper clothing (long-sleeved shirts and long pants that are tucked into sock cuffs), awareness of the seasons and habitat of ticks, and by applying repellent that contains 20% DEET or permethrin.

Prompt assessment for ticks and proper tick removal are also important.

A There is no vaccine for *R. rickettsii*, so active vaccination is not an option.

C Avoiding pets would not prevent infection, unless those pets have been exposed to the vector (which is not mentioned in this question).

D Avoidance of mouse droppings would be important for other zoonotic infections such as Hantavirus or leptospirosis, but not for *R. rickettsii*.

E Passive vaccination is also not available and would not be used for prevention in any case.

4. Correct: Nucleus (E)

R. rickettsii are obligate intracellular gram-negative coccobacilli. Upon infection of susceptible eukaryotic cells, these bacteria lyse the phagosomal membrane and escape to the cytosol. They replicate by binary fission in the host cell cytosol and nucleus. Most other intracellular bacterial pathogens replicate either within a membrane compartment such as a vacuole or phagosome, or in the cytosol. *R. rickettsii* are characteristically also able to replicate within the host cell nucleus.

A, B, C, D Virtually no intracellular pathogenic bacteria reside within the endoplasmic reticulum of host eukaryotic cells; however, there is some evidence for *Legionella pneumophila* and *Brucella* spp. to survive within ribosome-studded vacuoles. There is no evidence of bacterial growth in the Golgi apparatus or mitochondria of host eukaryotic cells. Lastly, many intracellular bacterial pathogens are able to halt phagosome–lysosome fusion, or survive within a phagolysosome; however, there are no pathogens that reside directly inside of a host cell lysosome.

5. Correct: Doxycycline (A)

The treatment for RMSF, no matter what the age of the patient, is doxycycline. Do not be fooled just because the patient is a child; doxycycline is used in children to treat RMSF and it is safe to do so. In smaller children, under 100 pounds, the dose is weight based, but otherwise the standard dose of 100 mg PO every 12 hours is used. The duration of therapy is at least 3 days past the resolution of fever and evidence of clinical improvement.

B, C, D, E None of the other antibiotics listed are used in the treatment of RMSF.

Keywords: Rocky Mountain spotted fever, *Rickettsia rickettsii*, tick, arthropod, *Dermacentor* spp., nucleus

Case 35

Adult Male with Worsening Shortness of Breath

A 49-year-old male presents to his primary care physician with increasing shortness of breath and a cough for the past 2 to 3 weeks. For the last week, he has noted a fever, increasing headaches, and weight loss. Social history indicates that the patient is a teacher, married in a monogamous relationship for the previous 26 years, and he enjoys fishing with his two teenaged sons. Past medical history is remarkable for a diagnosis 5 years earlier of chronic obstructive pulmonary disease (COPD) for which he has been taking inhaled steroids for the past several years. He has not traveled outside of the United States recently. Physical examination reveals a temperature of 38.7°C, blood pressure of 135/82 mmHg, and respiratory rate of 24 breaths/min. Decreased breath sounds are noted on auscultation. During the examination, the patient coughs and produces thick mucopurulent sputum, which is collected for laboratory testing. A chest radiograph is taken and reveals cavitation in the upper left lung with bilateral fluffy infiltrates. A purified protein derivative (PPD) skin test was negative. An acid-fast stain of the sputum is shown in the figure below. A sputum culture grew a similar organism that is also aerobic, weakly acid-fast, and gram-positive.

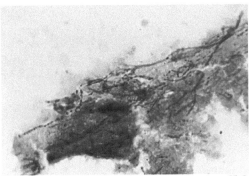

Image courtesy: CDC

Questions

1. Which of the following organisms is the most likely causative agent?

A. *Aspergillus fumigatus*

B. *Legionella pneumophila*

C. *Mycobacterium tuberculosis*

D. *Nocardia asteroides*

E. *Pseudomonas aeruginosa*

2. Which of the following is an important virulence factor of the most likely causative agent of this patient's infection?

A. Endotoxin

B. Exotoxin A

C. Granuloma formation

D. Resistance to phagocytosis

E. Urease production

3. Which of the following media would be used to culture the most likely causative agent in an aerobic environment in the laboratory?

A. Buffered charcoal yeast extract agar

B. MacConkey's agar

C. Mannitol salt agar

D. Tellurite blood agar

E. Thiosulphate-citrate-bile-sucrose (TCBS) agar

4. Which of the following is the most likely source of this patient's infection?

A. Arthropod bite

B. Endogenous

C. Ingestion of food

D. Ingestion of water

E. Inhalation

5. Given the patient's presentation and suspected infection what is the most important next test to obtain?

A. Blood cultures for acid-fast bacilli

B. Bronchioalveolar lavage

C. Computed tomography (CT) of the brain

D. Echocardiogram

E. Positron emission tomography (PET) scan

Answers and Explanations

1. Correct: *Nocardia asteroides* (D)

This case describes a patient with a respiratory infection. He has a predisposing risk to a more serious respiratory infection with a past medical history of COPD. It is also mentioned that he has not recently traveled outside of the United States, thereby limiting the possible causative agents to those more likely to be present in the United States. The figure shows a weakly acid-fast pleomorphic bacillus with branching filaments, indicating that the organism is likely positive to the modified acid-fast stain. *Nocardia* spp. contain some mycolic acid in their cell walls, causing these bacteria to stain acid-fast using the modified Kinyoun stain, which uses acid alcohol as the decolorizer instead of 1% sulfuric acid (which is used for traditional acid-fast staining procedures). The microscopic morphology also aids in determining the causative agent. *N. asteroides* typically appear as filamentous and branching rods that stain gram-positive on Gram stain. *Actinomyces* spp. look similar on Gram stain but are non–acid-fast, so those would be ruled out based on the acid-fast stain. Though *Nocardia* spp. appear fungi-like when viewed microscopically as well as macroscopically on media, they are taxonomically bacteria.

A, B, C, E With the exception of *Mycobacterium tuberculosis*, all of the other choices would stain non–acid-fast (blue) on the acid-fast stain and are therefore incorrect. *Aspergillus fumigatus* are fungi. *Haemophilus influenzae*, *Legionella pneumophila*, and *Pseudomonas aeruginosa* are gram-negative bacilli and do not display a filamentous morphology. Though *M. tuberculosis* are acid-fast, they are bacilli (acid-fast bacilli [AFB]) and are not filamentous.

2. Correct: Resistance to phagocytosis (D)

This case describes a patient with a respiratory tract infection caused by *Nocardia asteroides*. *Nocardia* spp. grow with a filamentous morphology in exponential phase growth, which aid in the resistance to phagocytosis. If the organisms are phagocytosed, phagosome–lysosome fusion is inhibited, thereby facilitating survival of *Nocardia* spp. within phagocytic cells. Furthermore, bacterial catalase and superoxide dismutase increase bacterial resistance to killing by host neutrophils.

A *Nocardia* spp. are gram-positive and therefore do not produce lipopolysaccharide (LPS) which is also known as endotoxin.

B *Nocardia* spp. are not known to produce any exotoxins during pathogenesis. Exotoxin A is produced by *P. aeruginosa*.

C Granuloma formation occurs during infections caused by *M. tuberculosis*.

E *Helicobacter pylori* produce urease during infection which facilitates survival of the organism in the low pH environment of the stomach.

3. Correct: Buffered charcoal yeast extract agar (A)

This case describes a patient with a *N. asteroides* respiratory infection. *Nocardia* spp. are aerobic bacteria that are able to be cultured on most routine bacterial, fungal, and mycobacterial culture media; however, many *Nocardia* spp. require up to 21 days for growth. Enrichment media is used to decrease the growth of other organisms and enhance the growth of *Nocardia* spp. Buffered charcoal yeast extract (media often used for isolation of *L. pneumophila*) and Thayer–Martin agar (media often used for isolation of *Neisseria* spp. or *H. influenzae*) are often used for isolation of *Nocardia* spp., however Löwenstein–Jensen media (media often used for isolation of *Mycobacterium* spp.) can also be used.

B MacConkey's agar is selective media used for the isolation of gram-negative enteric bacilli.

C Mannitol salt agar is selective and differential media that contains 7.5% NaCl and mannitol for isolation of most *Staphylococcus aureus* and *Micrococcus* spp. strains.

D Tellurite blood agar is selective medium for isolation of *Corynebacterium diphtheriae*.

E TCBS agar is selective medium used to isolate *Vibrio cholerae* and other *Vibrio* species from stool.

4. Correct: Inhalation (E)

This patient's respiratory tract infection is due to *N. asteroides*. *Nocardia* spp. are not normal human flora and are found worldwide in the environment, primarily soil and decaying matter. The organisms are also present in aquatic environments, can become air-borne and transmitted by inhalation to susceptible individuals. Because this patient is suffering from a respiratory infection, inhalation is the most likely route of infection.

A Because this patient enjoys fishing (an outdoor activity), it is feasible that he could have obtained the infection via an arthropod bite; however, there is no evidence for transmission of *N. asteroides* via arthropod vectors.

B *Nocardia* species are not normal flora; therefore endogenous transmission is not correct.

C, D In rare cases, *Nocardia* species are able to cause infection following ingestion of contaminated food or water; however, transmission via ingestion often results in gastrointestinal or systemic infection in individuals with multiple risk factors and a compromised immune system.

5. Correct: Computed tomography (CT) of the brain (C)

Nocardia spp. have a high propensity to disseminate to the central nervous system and can often cause brain abscess, even multiple brain abscesses. This patient, in addition to simply being at risk due to the *Nocardia* spp., has a symptom of headache that could be due to brain abscess. Knowing there is a brain abscess may change the selection of antibiotics toward those with enhanced penetration of the blood–brain barrier and will extend the duration of therapy to a minimum of 1 year. This knowledge may also suggest the addition of a third antibiotic or even possibly the need for surgical intervention.

A Blood cultures of *Nocardia* spp. are rarely positive.

B Given that we already have a positive sputum culture, there is no need to obtain a bronchoalveolar lavage (BAL) and would only be needed if sputum culture was unrevealing.

D Echocardiogram does not have a role in this case as *Nocardia* spp. rarely cause endocarditis.

E PET scan will not likely reveal any additional information in this case.

Keywords: *Nocardia asteroides*, COPD, nocardiosis, modified acid-fast, filamentous, buffered charcoal yeast extract

Case 36

Adult Female with Facial Pain

A 46-year-old female presents to the free clinic with complaints of a headache and facial pain. She is morbidly obese and says she hasn't seen a doctor since college. She says that she first noticed the headache 4 days earlier. She has lived in the Midwest her entire life. Physical examination shows swelling and redness along the right maxillary sinus, with pain upon palpation as well as significant proptosis of the right eye. Her temperature is 99.5°F, her blood pressure is 160/95 mmHg, and her respiratory rate is 22 breaths/min. She mentions that she had not eaten breakfast that morning, and so blood is obtained for a fasting glucose and other blood work. The fasting glucose is 240 mg/dL and hemoglobin (HgA1c) is 12.7%. The patient is sent to the local hospital and a computed tomography (CT) scan of the patient's head including dedicated sinus and orbit views is obtained. An otolaryngologist is called in to perform endoscopic examination of the sinuses where a black eschar is noted. The physician obtained a sample of the eschar from the patient's sinuses and sent it to the laboratory for culture. As soon as the physician is done with the endoscopic examination, treatment is immediately started. Three days later, cultures grew the organism, stained with lactophenol cotton blue, as seen in the figure below.

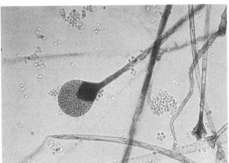

Image courtesy: CDC/ Dr. Lucille K. Georg

Questions

1. Which of the following organisms is the most likely causative agent?

A. *Cryptococcus neoformans*

B. *Mucor* spp.

C. *Sporothrix schenckii*

D. *Tinea versicolor*

E. *Trichophyton* spp.

2. Which of the following best describes a possible complication that may result from the infection with the most likely causative agent?

A. Blindness

B. Crepitus

C. Diffuse centripetal rash

D. Septicemia

E. Torticollis

3. Which of the following best describes the microscopic morphology of the most likely causative agent?

A. Weakly acid-fast beaded branching filaments

B. Broad-based budding yeast forms

C. Filamentous mold with broad, non-septate hyphae

D. Comma-shaped gram-negative rods

E. Gram-negative diplococci

4. Which of the following is an unusual but well-described risk factor for this infection?

A. Homeless shelter resident

B. Neonate in the neonatal intensive care unit (NICU)

C. Sickle cell anemia

D. Survival of a natural disaster

E. Previous urinary tract infection

5. What was the most appropriate treatment which was begun immediately after the endoscopy was complete?

A. Amphotericin B

B. Voriconazole

C. Deferasirox

D. Micafungin

E. Surgical debridement

Answers and Explanations

1. Correct: *Mucor* spp. (B)

This patient is suffering from a rhino-orbital mucormycosis infection. These infections are also sometimes called zygomycosis. Most infections are caused by fungi from the fungal taxonomic order *Mucorales*, including the genera *Mucor*, *Rhizopus*, and *Rhizomucor*. Diabetes is the single most significant risk factor for *Mucor*; it is also seen to a lesser extent in immunocompromised patients. Infection is rare in healthy immunocompetent individuals. The high fasting glucose and HgA1c are indicative of poor control of blood sugars. *Mucorales* fungi are able to proliferate in environments of high ketone or glucose concentrations. Furthermore, the figure shows a broad and non-septate fungal agent, indicative of *Mucor* or *Rhizopus* spp.

A *Cryptococcus neoformans* would more likely present as a respiratory or meningitis infection and would stain as encapsulated yeast.

C *Sporothrix schenckii* is the causative agent of rose handler's disease and would present as a cutaneous or subcutaneous infection and appear as dimorphic cigar-shaped yeast at 37°C or rosette conidia at 25°C

D *Tinea versicolor* (also known as pityriasis versicolor) is an infection caused by the fungi *Malassezia furfur* that results in pigmented macules and has a microscopic appearance described as spaghetti and meatballs.

E *Trichophyton* spp. are dermatophyte fungi that cause tinea (also known as ringworm) infections in the cutaneous layers of the skin.

2. Correct: Blindness (A)

This is a diabetic patient presenting with ketoacidosis and a mucormycosis infection. Diabetic ketoacidosis patients are at risk for mucormycosis, which often presents as a headache with a black eschar which can lead to an orbital, facial, or frontal lobe abscess. The most serious possible complication is death; however, involvement of the optic nerve may also lead to blindness. Given the extent of disease described it is almost certain she will lose her eye.

B Crepitus is sometimes seen in soft tissue infections involving *Clostridium perfringens*, or gas gangrene.

C The presence of a diffuse centripetal rash may be seen with infection due to viral etiologies such as Coxsackie A virus, herpes simplex virus, varicella-zoster, or vaccinia. Human immunodeficiency virus (HIV) is not a complication of any infection.

D Sepsis is the poisoning of blood by bacterial infection or toxin. Sepsis can be a complication of mucor infection but this would be in the context of gastrointestinal mucormycosis. In such an event, the fugus can invade the bowel causing perforation and bacterial translocation.

E Torticollis is a description for a flexion or extension of muscles of the neck and is not a complication of mucormycosis.

3. Correct: Filamentous mold with broad, non-septate hyphae (C)

The patient in this case has a mucormycosis infection that is affecting the orbit and causing proptosis. A predisposing factor of these infections is diabetes (and ketoacidosis), which is also described for this patient. The most likely causative agent would be fungi from the order *Mucorales*, such as *Mucor* or *Rhizopus* spp. *Mucor* spp. are fragile filamentous, nonbranching, and non-septated fungi that fragment easily and therefore must be handled carefully to allow for culture. Microscopically, the morphology can be described as broad, non-septate hyphae (to distinguish from *A. spergillus* spp. which are narrow).

A *Nocardia* spp. are weakly acid-fast bacilli that have a beaded branching filamentous appearance and are not the cause of the infection described here.

B Broad-based budding yeast describes *Blastomyces* spp., which are not the cause of this infection.

D, E *Vibrio* spp. are comma-shaped gram-negative rods that cause gastrointestinal

145

infections, and gram-negative diplococci such as *Neisseria* spp. are not shown in the figure.

4. Correct: Survival of a natural disaster (D)

This case describes a mucormycosis infection. It is thought that the largest risk factor for these infections is diabetes mellitus, particularly when ketoacidosis is involved. Other risk factors include cancer, transplantation, iron overload, AIDS, and injection drug use. These infections are also associated with natural disasters and combat. There have been cases of mucormycosis following tsunamis, tornados, and volcanic eruptions, as well as military personnel who sustained blast injuries.

A While malnutrition would be a risk factor, residents of homeless shelters should not be at greater risk than survivors of a natural disaster.

B A neonate in the NICU would not be at risk due to a lack of exposure to the fungal pathogens, which are present in the soil and outdoor environment.

C Sickle cell anemia patient would actually be less at risk for mucormycosis due to the fact that the fungal causative agent thrives in conditions of high iron.

E A previous urinary tract infection would have no effect on the risk of mucormycosis infection, unless the individuals also had other concurrent risk factors.

5. Correct: Surgical debridement (E)

The treatment of *Mucor* is to debride all the dead tissues and the mold until no more can be debrided. It is very similar to the treatment of necrotizing fasciitis where antibiotics are more of an adjuvant to treatment rather than the treatment itself. *Mucor* is nearly always fatal if not caught early enough and not debrided appropriately. In the case presented here, the patient will likely have her entire right eye and sinus network removed. If the infection is too widespread or invading the brain, it may be too late for debridement. When both eyes are affected, often the debridement will leave the skull unstable.

A, B, C, D Antifungals are used as an adjuvant to surgery and amphotericin B is the best studied. Voriconazole has no activity against *Mucor*. Although the newer azoles, posaconazole and isavuconazole, do have activity, they are generally not considered first line due to limited data on their use. Echinocandins like micafungin also have no activity against *Mucor* though there is some evidence that they are synergistic with amphotericin *B. Mucor* is an iron-loving mold and for many years it was thought that iron chelation would be a good addition to the treatment of *Mucor*. In the "DEFEAT Mucor" clinical trial of deferasirox for *Mucor*, the study was halted early due to a significant difference in mortality between the deferasirox chelator and the placebo. Unfortunately, the patients treated with deferasirox were the group which showed a significantly higher mortality.

Keywords: Mucormycosis, *Mucor* spp., *Rhizopus* spp., *Rhizomucor* spp., *Mucorales*, diabetes, ketoacidosis, non-septate hyphae

Case 37

Adult Female with Painful Rash

A 61-year-old female presents to her primary care physician in the summer with complaints of a mildly painful rash. She says that she first noticed the rash about a week earlier and that she believes she might be allergic to one of the flowers that she has been planting in her backyard. She mentions that she lives with her grandson who has a pet turtle that lives in a tank in his room, and that they also have a cat who roams the house freely and she changes the litter. Her past medical history is unremarkable and she is up-to-date on all recommended immunizations. Physical examination reveals two pustules with satellite lesions along the underside of the patient's left arm. Her temperature is 37°C, blood pressure is 128/84 mmHg, and heart rate is 70 bpm. A sample of fluid from the lesion is obtained and sent for Gram stain and culture onto Sabouraud's dextrose agar incubated at both 37°C and at room temperature. Microscopic examination of the Gram stain is shown in the figure below.

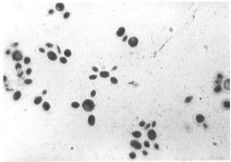

Image courtesy: CDC/ Dr. Lucille K. Georg

Questions

1. Which of the following organisms is the most likely causative agent?

A. *Bartonella henselae*

B. *Salmonella agbeni*

C. *Toxoplasma gondii*

D. *Histoplasma capsulatum*

E. *Sporothrix schenckii*

2. For the most likely causative agent, what is the microscopic morphology that one would expect from the organism cultivated at 25°C?

A. Cigar-shaped budding yeast

B. Gram-negative bacilli

C. Gram-positive cocci

D. A crescent-shaped protozoa

E. Rosette pattern of conidia on conidiophore

3. Which of the following best describes the cell wall of the most likely causative agent?

A. Layer of cellulose

B. Layer of chitin

C. Outer membrane containing lipo-oligosaccharide (LOS)

D. Outer membrane containing lipopolysaccharide (LPS)

E. Thick peptidoglycan layer

4. Which of the following is the most likely source of this patient's infection?

A. Cat

B. Garden plants

C. Mosquitoes

D. Ticks

E. Turtle in the house

5. What is the most appropriate treatment for this infection?

A. Itraconazole

B. Amphotericin B

C. Pyrimethamine

D. Azithromycin

E. No treatment is needed; it will resolve on its own

Answers and Explanations

1. Correct: *Sporothrix schenckii* (E)

This case describes a patient with "rose handler's disease" or sporotrichosis, caused by the fungi *Sporothrix schenckii*. It is a subacute or chronic infection that causes a localized nodule that drains to the lymphatics. The infection often involves the cutaneous or subcutaneous tissues of the arms or legs following inoculation of the organism from the soil through the skin. At risk are any individuals who are involved with landscaping, gardening, tree farming, or other outdoor activities that may result in breaks in the skin with soil present. Furthermore, the Gram stain image shows cigar-shaped budding yeast, characteristic of the dimorphic fungi *S. schenckii*, when grown at 37°C (body temperature).

A *Bartonella henselae* is the causative agent of cat-scratch disease and are small pleomorphic gram-negative bacilli-shaped bacteria.

B *Salmonella agbeni* is a gram-negative bacterium causing gastrointestinal illness, transmitted by ingestion of contaminated food or water or handling reptiles.

C *Toxoplasma gondii* is a parasite carried in cat feces, but the infection it causes primarily affects immunosuppressed patients and the typical symptoms do not match this case.

D *Histoplasma capsulatum* causes respiratory infections in endemic areas, are transmitted from bat and bird fecal matter, and are small yeast cells when cultivated at 37°C.

2. Correct: Rosette pattern of conidia on conidiophore (E)

This patient is infected with *S. schenckii*. *S. schenckii* exhibit thermal dimorphism. These fungi are cigar-shaped budding yeast at 37°C and have a characteristic rosette pattern of conidia on conidiophore at 25°C

A This question is asking about the morphology at 25°C; therefore, cigar-shaped

budding yeast (such as those seen in the figure) is an incorrect answer.

B, C *S. schenckii* are fungi and not bacteria; therefore, gram-negative bacilli and gram-positive cocci are incorrect answers.

D A crescent-shaped protozoa is the description of *T. gondii*.

3. Correct: Layer of chitin (B)

This case describes a patient infected with the fungus *S. schenckii*. therefore, this question is asking about the composition of a typical fungal cell wall (eukaryote). Fungal membranes are usually stabilized with ergosterol. The surrounding cell wall is typically composed of chitin. Plant (eukaryote) cell walls contain cellulose.

A, C, D, E The other answer choices describe bacterial (prokaryote) cell walls: gram-positive bacterial cell walls are composed of a thick peptidoglycan layer; gram-negative cell walls are composed of a thin peptidoglycan layer and an outer membrane. Most gram-negative outer membranes contain LPS but some contain LOS, for example *Neisseria* spp. and *Haemophilus* spp.

4. Correct: Garden plants (B)

This patient is infected with the fungus *S. schenckii*. This infection is also known as rose handler's disease due to the typical route of infection: a gardener who becomes infected while pruning rose bushes and is pricked by a thorn. The break in the skin allows the fungi to enter the body from the soil or dust on the exterior of the plants. In the case of this patient, the source of the infection was from her garden plants.

A, C, D, E, *S. schenckii* are not a part of normal human flora, therefore, endogenous transmission is unlikely. Though this patient was likely exposed to both mosquitoes and ticks while tending to her garden, *S. schenckii* are not transmitted by arthropod bites. It is mentioned that the patient's grandson owns a turtle. Turtles are commonly a source of *Salmonella* spp. Infections; however there is no evidence of transmission of *S. schenckii*. There is, however, evidence of transmission of *S. schenckii* by cats and armadillos who carry soil on their claws and may transmit the organism to humans through a scratch.

5. Correct: Itraconazole (A)

The most appropriate treatment for mild cutaneous sporotrichosis is itraconazole.

B Amphotericin B would be used for severe sporotrichosis or disseminated sporotrichosis.

C Pyrimethamine is the treatment for toxoplasmosis.

D Azithromycin is often used for severe cat-scratch disease.

E In general, while the infection is not life threatening, it will take several months of antifungals to resolve.

Keywords: *Sporothrix schenckii*, rose-handlers disease, dimorphic, fungi, cigar-shaped, rosette conidia

Case 38

Adult Female with Headache and Confusion

A 26-year-old female is brought to the emergency room by her husband. For the past several days, she has had a fever, chills, and a headache, and this morning she became confused and less responsive, so her husband brought her to the hospital. The patient was intubated for airway protection and a Foley catheter was placed. Dark-colored urine was seen draining from the catheter. The patient was unresponsive, but her husband noted a past medical history of immune thrombocytopenic purpura as a teenager, which was treated with steroids and eventually with a splenectomy at age 19 when it was refractory to steroid treatment. The patient had no other medical problems and was taking no medications at the time of admission. She works as an advertising executive and has had no sick contacts. The couple has been married for 3 years and they have no children. They are sexually active and were using condoms until the past 3 months when they began trying to have a baby. The patient's husband says that they are monogamous, but then admits that he suspects she might have had an affair with a man they met while camping. They have no pets and she has no unusual exposures. They have not travelled outside of the country since their honeymoon to Bali 3 years ago, but they did go to upstate New York 2 weeks prior for a camping trip.

On examination, the patient is intubated and sedated, not responsive to questions or commands. Her eye examination notes scleral icterus and there is a notable jaundice to the skin. A scar from the prior splenectomy is noted, but otherwise her examination is normal. Blood was drawn and sent to the laboratory for evaluation. Her hematocrit is 25 percent, platelet count is 50,000/mL, and white blood cell (WBC) count is 12,000 cells/mm³. Her serum lactate dehydrogenase is 450 units/L and total bilirubin is 13 umol/L. The remainder of her liver function tests and blood urea nitrogen (BUN)/creatinine are normal. A microscopic evaluation by thin blood smear was done as shown in the figure below.

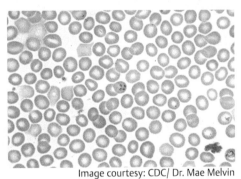

Image courtesy: CDC/ Dr. Mae Melvin

Questions

1. Which of the following organisms is most likely responsible for this patient's symptoms?

A. *Babesia microti*

B. *Borrelia burgdorferi*

C. *Coxiella burnetii*

D. *Plasmodium falciparum*

E. *Rickettsia rickettsii*

2. Which of the following tests is the diagnostic standard for identifying the causative organism?

A. Clinical signs and symptoms

B. Immunofluorescent antibody

C. Microscopy

D. Polymerase chain reaction (PCR)

E. Western blot

3. Which of the following is a stereotypic indication of this organism?

A. Band form

B. Maltese cross form

C. Proglottid form

D. Reticulate body form

E. Ring form

4. Which of the following is most likely the mode of transmission of this patient's infection?

A. Ingestion of contaminated water

B. Inhalation of contaminated air

C. Mosquito bite

D. Sexual contact

E. Tick bite

5. What is the most appropriate initial treatment for this patient?

A. Artemether–lumefantrine

B. Clindamycin and quinine

C. Doxycycline

D. Supportive care only

E. Vancomycin and piperacillin–tazobactam

Answers and Explanations

1. Correct: *Babesia microti* (A)

This is a case of babesiosis caused by the apicomplexan parasite *Babesia* spp., of which there are multiple species that cause human disease, but the most common in the United States is *Babesia microti*. *Babesia* spp., reproduce asexually in the erythrocytes of their mammalian host but sexually reproduce in the arthropod vector. In the United States, the infection is spread by the deer tick (*Ixodes scapularis*) which also spreads Lyme disease and anaplasmosis. Patients often do not report a tick bite as this tick is small and often goes unnoticed. In addition to tick-borne cases, transfusion-related cases have been reported. There is a range of infection manifestations from asymptomatic to severe disease with most cases being asymptomatic or mild and self-limited but occasionally being moderate (requiring treatment) or even severe and life threatening. Severe disease primarily occurs in those that are asplenic but can occur in other immunosuppressed patients including those with HIV or even rarely in immunocompetent patients. Asplenic patients are at high risk for severe disease because without the spleen, infected red blood cells cannot be removed from circulation and the percentage of infected cells increases. The location of travel in this case gives indication of potential infectious cause of these symptoms and the potential for vector-borne transmission while camping should also be considered.

B, C, D, E *Plasmodium falciparum*, the causative agent of malaria, would not be expected to be transmitted in New York. Transmission of *Coxiella* spp., the causative agent of Q fever, would be more associated with domestic farming locales. *Rickettsia* spp., infections can cause spotted fevers including the more severe Rocky Mountain spotted fever. This infection is transmitted rarely in New York and would not necessarily be the first choice but should

considered in the differential. *Borrelia* spp., the causative agent of Lyme disease, should be considered, but the clinical situation given is not consistent with Lyme disease.

2. Correct: Microscopy (C)

The diagnostic gold standard for acute babesiosis is the microscopic evaluation of a blood smear. It takes an experienced individual looking at many thin smear slides to confirm *Babesia* spp. in low level parasitemia. Ring forms may be commonly seen and hard to distinguish from *Plasmodium* spp., however, the Maltese cross form where merozoites are arranged in tetrads is pathognomonic for *Babesia* spp. infection. It is important that a quick diagnosis be established due to the severity of the infection in this case.

A Clinical signs and symptoms are not sufficient for diagnosis as symptoms are similar to the other organisms listed. Additionally, many infections are asymptomatic.

B Immunofluorescent antibody testing is available for *Babesia* spp. infection but it is not considered the standard. Negative IFA results would require additional molecular testing.

D Molecular testing with PCR is sometimes helpful in low levels of *Babesia* spp. parasitemia but is not commonly available.

E Serology and Western blot have no utility in diagnosing an acute babesiosis, but they are used for diagnosis of Lyme disease.

3. Correct: Maltese cross form (B)

The stereotypic marker observed when evaluating blood smears is the Maltese cross band form as shown in the figure. This characteristic image is caused by a tetrad of parasites within the same blood cell. This form is transient but can be observed in an acute infection during the merozoite phase in the infected erythrocyte. It can be confused with the ring form of *P. falciparum*.

A A band form describes a mature trophozoite of *Plasmodium malariae*.

C Proglottids are worm segments and would be seen in fecal specimens in helminth infections

D, E A reticulate body form is the internalized replicative form for chlamydial infection. This infection occurs in squamous epithelia cells and not in erythrocytes.

4. Correct: Tick bite (E)

Babesia spp. is transmitted by a tick bite from primarily the deer tick, *I. scapularis*. The most common reservoir for *B. microti* is the white-footed mouse (*Peromyscus leucopus*). Humans are an incidental host. Transmission occurs most often in Northeast and upper Midwest regions of the United States. It is the nymph stage of the tick that is responsible for transmission when taking a blood meal. Transmission events to humans occur most often in wooded or grassy areas during the spring and summer months.

A *Babesia* spp. do not survive for long periods of time in contaminated water; this is the location of *Giardia* and other organisms.

B This parasite is not transmitted via contaminated air.

C Unlike *Plasmodium* spp., *Babesia* spp. is not transmitted by mosquito.

D *Babesia* spp. has not been reported to be transmitted via sexual contact.

5. Correct: Clindamycin and quinine (B)

The standard treatment for severe *Babesia* spp. infection is intravenous (IV) clindamycin and oral quinine (IV quinine is no longer available in the United States). Another option for treatment is IV azithromycin plus oral atovaquone. This regimen is often used for the treatment of mild-to-moderate babesiosis but is less well studied in severe babesiosis infections, though some sources place it first line in therapy. Current guidelines recommend clindamycin and quinine as first-line treatment. In an asplenic patient, it is important to determine the percentage of red blood cells which are infected (parasitemia) as an exchange transfusion is often required in patients with a parasitemia of greater than or equal to 10 percent, and the treatment success can be tracked by reduction of the parasite burden. Failures of therapy and relapses have been seen in patients in whom treatment is stopped before resolution of the parasitemia.

A, C, D, E Doxycycline is used to treat several tick-borne diseases including Lyme disease and anaplasmosis, also carried by the deer tick and *Rickettsia* infection, carried by the dog tick. Doxycycline is also used to treat Q fever caused by *Coxiella* spp. However, doxycycline has no role in treating babesiosis. Artemether–lumefantrine is used to treat malaria. Vancomycin and piperacillin–tazobactam are often used together to empirically treat a septic patient but have no role in treating *Babesia* spp. infections. Supportive care would never be used in severe babesiosis or in an asplenic patient with babesiosis. Some physicians favor supportive care for mild cases of the disease, but current guidelines recommend treating all patients with active, symptomatic babesiosis.

Keywords: Parasite, babesiosis, immunocompromised, blood, insect vector, clindamycin, quinine

Case 39

Adult Male with Painful, Swollen Lymph Nodes

An 18-year-old male presents to the hospital with 24 hours of severely swollen, painful cervical lymph nodes. He reports he has pain with swallowing, and he can no longer swallow solids or liquids. He relates that for the past 5 days he has had a fever up to 101°F, chills, night sweats, headaches, muscle aches, and fatigue. Three days prior he developed a rash. The patient has no significant past medical history, is not on any medications, and has no known allergies. He is up-to-date on immunizations and recently had a battery of extra immunizations from a travel clinic prior to a trip to Africa he took with his family about a month ago. He returned from Africa 2 weeks ago. While in Africa, he ate native foods including uncooked fruit and vegetables and he drank local water. He stayed mostly in resorts but did go on a safari where he stayed in tents and was able to handle smaller captive native animals. He reports an unprotected sexual encounter with a native woman while he was there.

On examination, he is alert but ill-appearing. His vital signs are: temperature 101.3°F, blood pressure (BP) 120/75 mmHg, heart rate (HR) 116 bpm, and respiratory rate (RR) 24 breaths/min. He has numerous flat red macules over the face, trunk, and extremities, including the palms of the hands (see figure below) and soles of the feet, which he reports had then spread over his entire body. There are also several papules, vesicles, and pustules within the patient's oral cavity. He has a bull-neck appearance with several 2 to 3 cm tender palpable nodes bilaterally. His lungs are clear and he has no stridor. Heart is tachycardic but with a normal rhythm. The rest of the examination is essentially normal.

His white blood cell (WBC) count is 17×10^6 cells/μL, but the remainder of his laboratories is normal.

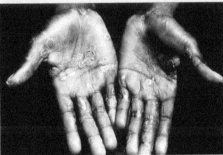

Image courtesy: CDC/ Brian W.J. Mahy

Questions

1. Which of the following is the mostly likely etiology of this infection?

A. Coxsackie A virus

B. Measles virus

C. Monkeypox virus

D. *Neisseria gonorrhoeae*

E. Varicella-zoster virus

2. Which of the following best describes the etiologic agent?

A. A double-stranded DNA virus

B. A single-stranded DNA virus

C. A gram-negative diplococcus

D. A single-stranded RNA virus

E. A retrovirus

3. Which of the following is the most likely source of this infection?

A. Animal exposure in Africa

B. Natural water in Africa

C. Sexual transmission

D. A source not related to the African trip

E. Uncooked fruit and vegetables in Africa

4. Electron microscopy of tissue from the lesions will most likely show which of the following?

A. Bean-shaped bacteria

B. Brick-like virions

C. Helical virions

D. Icosahedral virions

E. Spherical virions

5. The most appropriate therapy for this patient is which of the following?

A. Vaccination with smallpox vaccine

B. Intravenous immunoglobulin (IVIg)

C. Cidofovir

D. Ceftriaxone

E. Supportive care

Answers and Explanations

1. Correct: Monkeypox virus (C)

This case describes a probable episode of monkeypox. There are several clues to suggest this and differentiate it from the other choices. Monkeypox is endemic in parts of Africa and sporadic in many other parts. The incubation period is 5 to 21 days, and the illness begins with a prodrome that can include fever, headache, myalgias, swollen lymph nodes, chills, and fatigue. Generally, the rash begins 1 to 3 days after the onset of fever which progresses through multiple stages starting with macules then papules, vesicles, pustules, and finally scabbing over. The illness can last up to a month. The severe lymphadenopathy is one factor that distinguishes monkeypox from smallpox which does not typically have lymphadenopathy.

A Coxsackie A virus is unlikely as the rash is comprised of a blister-type rash that is contained to the mouth, palms of the hand, and soles of the feet, unlike that described in this case.

B While measles rash does initiate at the head with Koplik's spots often evident in the mouth, the rash progresses toward the trunk and extremities and does not begin on the hands and feet. The history of the spread of this rash makes measles less likely.

D *Neisseria gonorrhoeae* is unlikely as disseminated gonorrhea will generally start with a urethritis which this patient did not have, and the rash is maculopapular, but not generally vesicular.

E Varicella-zoster virus is unlikely as the patient was up-to-date on his immunizations. This would include varicella zoster. While it is possible to have failed immunity or break-through infection, this is less likely. In addition, the rash of chickenpox usually has many different types of lesions with some crusting over within 24 hours and otherwise is primarily vesicular and rarely on the palms and soles.

2. Correct: A double-stranded DNA virus (A)

The etiologic agent of monkeypox is monkeypox virus which is one of the pox viruses of the *Poxviridae* family. It is a double-stranded DNA virus.

B The choice of single-stranded DNA virus is incorrect; most of these types of viruses are not human pathogens but include several bacteriophages, and other viruses which tend to infect microorganisms though there are some that do infect vertebrate animals.

C Gram-negative diplococcus is incorrect and would indicate an infection such as gonorrhea.

D Single-stranded RNA virus is incorrect; many viruses fall into this category and can be positive sense including hepatitis C virus, dengue virus, corona virus, and rhinovirus; or negative sense including Ebola virus, measles, mumps, and rabies.

E Retrovirus is incorrect; retroviruses are a specific form of positive-sense RNA virus which uses a DNA intermediate in its replication cycle. HIV is the archetypical example of a retrovirus.

3. Correct: Animal exposure in Africa (A)

Monkeypox is generally considered a zoonotic disease and the primary hosts are African rodents that the patient likely was exposed to on the safari where he was able to handle small captive native animals. Transmission from animals can occur when a person is exposed to contaminated material or body fluids from the animal, and the virus can enter via the respiratory tract, mucous membranes, or a break in the skin such as a bite or scratch. Human-to-human transmission is possible but less common.

B Natural water in Africa can cause such diseases as amebic dysentery, hepatitis A, cholera, and typhoid.

C Sexual transmission can lead to infection by HIV and gonorrhea as well as syphilis, chlamydia, and numerous other sexually transmitted infections (STIs).

D Infections not related to the African trip might include infectious mononucleosis and chickenpox.

E Uncooked fruit and vegetables are a common way various gastrointestinal (GI) pathogens spread, including *Escherichia coli*, *Salmonella*, and various intestinal parasites.

4. Correct: Brick-like virions (B)

Electron microscopy is frequently a significant diagnostic modality in monkeypox, though it cannot distinguish it from other poxviruses. The typical description of monkeypox virus is brick shaped with lateral bodies and a central core.

A Bean-shaped bacteria is a description associated with *N. gonorrhoeae*, but generally, bacteria are too large to view via electron microscopy.

C Helical virions include Ebola virus and rabies virus.

D Icosahedral virions include common viruses such as adenovirus and rhinovirus.

E Spherical virions are generally enveloped icosahedral viral particles where the envelope makes the virion appear more spherical and includes HIV.

5. Correct: Supportive care (E)

Unfortunately, there is no proven therapy for monkeypox, and supportive care is generally the only treatment.

A Older data from Africa suggest smallpox vaccine may prevent monkeypox as well, but this vaccine is generally no longer available. The Centers for Disease Control and Prevention (CDC) has considered its use for outbreaks of monkeypox.

B IVIg, specifically Vaccinia immune globulin has also been suggested for use in monkeypox, but there are again no data.

C Cidofovir has in vitro activity and has shown activity in animal models, but there are no data in humans.

D Ceftriaxone has no activity against viruses, but it could be used in the treatment of gonorrhea, though emerging resistance is limiting its use there.

Keywords: Monkeypox, double stranded DNA, animal exposure, pox virus

Case 40

Toddler with High Fever and Upper Respiratory Symptoms

A 14-month-old girl is brought to urgent care with a 3-day history of high fever, cough, and runny nose. Upon physical examination, the physician notes small white spots on the inside of the child's mouth (see figure below) and catarrhal inflammation within the nose. The child also shows signs of conjunctivitis in the right eye. The mother reports that the child is lethargic and refuses to eat. The child attends a private day care and is not current with vaccinations. The family owns a cat and spends a lot of time outdoors.

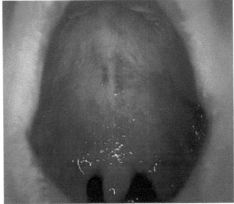

Image courtesy: CDC/ Heinz F. Eichenwald

Questions

1. Which of the following organisms is the most probable cause of these symptoms?

A. Adenovirus

B. Epstein–Barr virus

C. Measles virus

D. *Streptococcus pneumoniae*

E. *Streptococcus pyogenes*

2. Which of the following signs is most likely to manifest in this patient within the next 3 days?

A. Diarrhea

B. Reddish-brown rash

C. Stiff neck

D. Vomiting

E. Desquamation

3. What is the mode of transmission for this infection?

A. Animal

B. Arthropod-borne

C. Droplet

D. Fecal–oral

E. Skin-to-skin contact

4. Which of the following is the usual means for diagnosing this infection?

A. Clinical signs

B. Immunoglobulin G (IgG) avidity testing

C. Plaque reduction neutralization assay

D. Reverse transcription polymerase chain reaction (RT-PCR)

E. Biopsy

5. At the age of 10, this patient develops mood swings that last for approximately 6 months and then starts to have uncontrolled jerking motions. She is seen by a neurologist who tells her parents that this is a rare complication of the infection that the girl had at the age of 14 months. Which of the following best describes this complication?

A. PANDAS

B. MELAS

C. MERRF

D. SSPE

E. PML

Answers and Explanations

1. Correct: Measles virus (C)

This is a case of measles (formerly known as rubeola) caused by the negative sense single-stranded RNA measles virus of the *Paramyxoviridae* family. The Koplik spots, bluish-white spots on a red background, noted on the mucosa of the oral cavity (seen in the figure) along with the fever, cough, and runny nose indicate measles. Additionally, conjunctivitis can occur which presents as the classic triad conjunctivitis, inflammation of the membranes of the nose (coryza).

A, B, D, E None of the other answer choices listed result in this group of clinical symptoms, and the Koplik spots are unique to measles infection.

2. Correct: Reddish-brown rash (B)

Measles presents after 2 to 3 days of fever with a reddish-Brown rash that extends across the entire body. It usually begins at the head and proceeds downward to the trunk, arms, legs, and feet. The rash lasts approximately a week after the first appearance.

A, C, D, E Measles typically does not present with gastrointestinal (GI) symptoms such as diarrhea or vomiting. Desquamation is not typically seen with measles; it is seen in cases of toxic shock syndrome. While measles can cause an encephalopathy (subacute sclerosing panencephalitis), it does not typically cause meningitis, and encephalopathy is rare.

3. Correct: Droplet (C)

Measles virus is spread person-to-person by coughing and sneezing. The airborne virus is thought to infect alveolar macrophages in the airway and then spreads to other lymphocytic cells in lymphatic organs.

A, B, D, E There is no known animal or insect reservoir for measles virus. This virus is not transmitted via the fecal–oral route, or by skin-to-skin contact.

4. Correct: Clinical signs (A)

The usual method of diagnosing measles is by clinical signs such as Koplik's spots and the measles rash. Measles is a routine vaccination in many countries and as a result, clinical cases are uncommon in those countries. In the United States, measles is a routine vaccination (measles, mumps, and rubella [MMR]), and so cases are rare, and the signs are usually caused by other rash-causing illnesses. When testing is done, it is by serological testing and IgM detection within the first few days of the illness. However, given the reduction in compliance with vaccination espoused by some parents, measles has seen a resurgence throughout the world.

B, C, D, E IgG avidity testing, plaque reduction neutralization assay, RT-PCR, and biopsy are not routinely utilized for diagnosis of measles.

5. Correct: SSPE (D)

A rare complication of measles infection is subacute sclerosing panencephalitis (SSPE), which is rare in the United States but during outbreaks has been as high as 11 cases in 100,000 patients. It usually occurs 7 to 10 years after the initial infection and seems to be more common in people infected prior to the age of 2. It is a progressive neurological disease which is generally fatal within 3 years. It has four stages: Stage 1 includes mood swings, personality changes, and depression. There may be associated fever and headaches. Stage 2 includes uncontrolled jerking movements and muscle spasms. This can be accompanied by vision loss, dementia, and seizures. In stage 3, the jerking motions become writhing and rigidity. Stage 4 includes autonomic dysfunction, coma, and death.

A PANDAS is pediatric autoimmune neuropsychiatric disorders associated with streptococcal infections and are tic disorders and obsessive-compulsive disorder linked to group A *Streptococcus* infection.

B MELAS is mitochondrial encephalomyopathy, lactic acidosis, and stroke-like episodes which is a disease caused by mutations in

161

the mitochondrial genome and associated in childhood with muscle weakness, pain, recurrent headaches and seizures, and eventually strokes in adult years.

C MERRF is myoclonic epilepsy with ragged red fibers, another disease linked to mutations in the mitochondrial genome which causes a progressive form of myoclonic epilepsy.

E PML is progressive multifocal leukoencephalopathy which is caused by John Cunningham (JC) virus in immunosuppressed patients and leads to inflammation and demyelination of the white matter causing progressive weakness, visual changes, speech difficulty, loss of coordination, seizures, and personality changes.

Keywords: Enanthem, respiratory infection, vaccination, pediatric, measles, rubeola

Case 41

Adult Female with Febrile Illness

A physician on a medical mission in Sierra Leone assessed a 31-year-old female patient presenting with an acute illness of approximately 1-week duration. She felt febrile though he did not take her temperature; she noted extreme fatigue and achiness for the first few days and then developed abdominal pain, nausea, and diarrhea for the last 3 days. Upon examination, the patient was found to have a fever of 38.5°C, a blood pressure (BP) of 95/60 mmHg, a heart rate of 120 bpm, and a respiratory rate of 26 breaths/min. She looked ill and had dry mucous membranes and a notable maculopapular rash on the arms and torso which was nonpruritic. The patient was admitted to the hospital and given empiric malaria treatment. Routine laboratories showed leukopenia, thrombocytopenia, elevated creatinine, elevated liver enzymes, as well as an elevated prothrombin time and international normalized ratio PT/INR. A rapid malaria test was ordered and the result was negative. Blood was drawn and sent to the national laboratory where it was determined the genome of the infectious agent was single-stranded negative sense RNA. The following day, the patient complained of worsening abdominal pain and developed hematochezia, hematuria, and hematemesis. She declined rapidly with diminishing urine output and decreasing level of consciousness and proceeded to expiration in the next 24 hours.

Questions

1. Which of the following pathogens is most likely the cause of the symptoms in this patient?

A. Ebola virus

B. Lassa fever virus

C. *Plasmodium falciparum*

D. *Salmonella enterica typhi*

E. Yellow fever virus

2. Which of the following is the best method for confirmation of acute infection?

A. Culture of pathogen

B. Immunoglobulin G (IgG) antibody detection

C. Immunohistochemistry

D. Rapid test

E. Reverse transcriptase polymerase chain reaction (RT-PCR) nucleic acid detection

3. What is the mostly likely transmission event that caused this infection?

A. Animal bite

B. Blood and body fluid

C. Contaminated food

D. Insect vector

E. Rodent excrement

4. With consistent daily cleaning and infection control practices, what is the maximum time contaminated surfaces within the patient care environment could remain infectious and transmissible with the causative pathogen?

A. Two hours

B. Twenty-four hours

C. One week

D. One month

E. Indefinitely

5. Which of the following is the most appropriate treatment for this patient?

A. Artesunate

B. Cidofovir

C. Ciprofloxacin

D. Intravenous immunoglobulin (IVIg)

E. Supportive care and hydration

Answers and Explanations

1. Correct: Ebola virus (A)

This is a case of Ebola virus infection. Ebola virus is transmitted from contaminated objects and body fluids of infected people. Ebola should be considered in the differential not only due to presentation but also because of the location. West Central Africa has been the site of a large multinational outbreak of Ebola virus infection in recent years. Determination of travel to these areas should also be considered for patients who present with similar symptoms when identified domestically in the United States. Ebola may be misdiagnosed as early symptoms are not specific. Other hemorrhagic fevers should be considered in the differential and would be ruled out by RT-PCR and IgM enzyme-linked immunosorbent assay (ELISA) detection. Ebola virus is a member of the *Filoviridae* family. There are five viral species, four of which cause disease in humans and originate in Africa: Zaire ebolavirus, Sudan ebolavirus, Taï Forest ebolavirus, and Bundibugyo ebolavirus. A transmission electron microscopy (TEM) of Ebola virus is shown in the following figure.

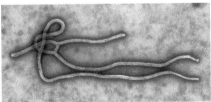

Image courtesy: CDC/ Cynthia Goldsmith

B Lassa Fever virus has a long negative sense and short ambisense RNA genome.
C Marlaria, because of the fever, chills, and headaches along with gastrointestinal symptoms, is often the first considered in a misdiagnosis. Diagnosis of malaria can be done in the field with rapid diagnostic testing, but the gold standard is microscopy of thick and thin blood films looking for parasites.

D *Salmonella* does not have an RNA genome. Typhoid fever has additional symptoms of rose spot rash appearing on the anterior trunk and jaundice.
E Yellow Fever virus has a single-stranded positive sense RNA genome.

2. Correct: Reverse transcriptase polymerase chain reaction (RT-PCR) nucleic acid detection (E)

RT-PCR is the best method for detection of acute infection. Detection of acute infection should occur within 3 to 10 days of the presentation of symptoms, and RT-PCR along with IgM ELISA are best suited for acute detection. In the severe hemorrhagic stage, patients often die before an immune response can be detected making RT-PCR most valuable.
A, B, C, D Culture of the virus is dangerous and requires biosafety level 4 containment; these types of facilities are infrequent in most countries, and there are currently only eight such laboratories in the United States. Detection of IgG is used in the recovery phase of the illness. Immunohistochemistry is used in the detection of virus from tissues of deceased patients. While rapid testing for Ebola is available and the first test has been recently approved by the U.S. FDA, this is for presumptive diagnosis and not confirmatory testing at this time.

3. Correct: Blood and body fluid (B)

Ebola virus infects nonhuman primates as well as humans and has been found to cause an asymptomatic infection in fruit bats. It is not certain how the virus enters the human population, but it is believed to be a zoonotic infection arising from butchering and eating bush meat or handling infected bats. Most infections occur because of a transmission of blood and body fluids from an infected individual to those who are caring for them. The virus is often transmitted by contaminated objects like bedding. In the 2014 West African outbreak, a great deal of spread occurred from the dead to people performing funeral rites involving washing of the body. Additionally, sexual transmission has been reported.

A, C, D, E The virus is not transmitted by arthropod vector or by contaminated food. The virus could be transmitted via the bite of an infected animal but it is thought that this is a rare transmission event. Rodent feces have not been identified as a vehicle for transmission.

4. Correct: Twenty-four hours (B)

Ebola is an enveloped RNA virus with the capsid morphology having a worm-like appearance (see figure). Even if a virus may not be easily treated, an enveloped virus is more sensitive to decontamination. Enveloped viruses in general degrade easily due to environmental conditions such as drying and ultraviolet radiation. However, Ebola can remain infectious on a contaminated surface for up to 24 hours depending on humidity as determined by the study by Bausch et al. in blood and body fluid spills as well as damp contaminated laundry, Ebola may remain infectious in reduced viral concentrations for several days. It has recently been understood that the virus is present for many months in ocular fluid and semen samples from individuals who have recovered from Ebola illness.

A Virus remains infectious and transmissible well beyond two hours on a contaminated surface although the risk is low.

C Ebola may remain infectious in reduced viral concentrations for several days, but limiting concentrations further reduce likelihood of transmission.

D, E The time frames of one month to indefinite are not reported for transmission.

5. Correct: Supportive care and hydration (E)

Although there are many experimental therapies in development for the treatment of Ebola virus infection, the only accepted treatment is supportive care with particular attention to fluid and electrolyte replacement.

A, B, C, D Artesunate is a treatment used for malaria infections. Because this is a viral infection, antibiotics such as ciprofloxacin are useless. Therapy for support of the immune system, such as IVIg, has not been found to be effective to date. Research into the development of antiviral therapy specific for the treatment of Ebola infection is ongoing, but cidofovir does not have activity against Ebola.

Keywords: Parasite, bloodborne pathogen, select agent, malaria, Ebola virus

Case 42

Agitated Male with Rapid Progression to Coma

A 34-year-old male was brought to the emergency department by a friend with signs of fever, pharyngeal spasms, confusion, and agitation. The friend reports that the patient has been ill on and off for the past month when he returned from a mission trip to Mexico with flu-like symptoms that lasted for about a week and then resolved. More recently, he complained of headache and insomnia. An electroencephalogram showed diffuse abnormalities indicative of encephalopathy. The patient was admitted to the hospital and within 24 hours fell into a coma. The patient remained on life support for another 10 days before succumbing to the infection. A postmortem biopsy of the cerebellum tissue is shown in the figure below.

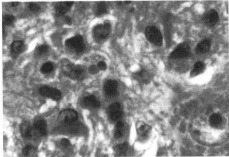

Image courtesy: CDC/ Dr. Daniel P. Perl

Questions

1. Which of the following organisms is most likely the cause of this patient's death?

A. *Clostridium tetani*

B. Herpes simplex virus

C. Rabies virus

D. *Toxoplasma gondii*

E. West Nile virus

2. Which of the following pathologies is indicative of this infection in a postmortem evaluation of tissue?

A. Bielschowsky bodies

B. Cowdry type A bodies

C. Cowdry type B bodies

D. Negri bodies

E. Paschen bodies

3. Which of the following scenarios is most probable for transmission of this organism?

A. Animal bite

B. Cat litter box

C. Mosquito bite

D. Sexual

E. Unwashed wound

4. Which of the following is most useful in the antemortem diagnosis of this infection?

A. Clinical signs

B. Culture

C. Western blot

D. Polymerase chain reaction (PCR)

E. Skin biopsy

5. If the patient had seen a doctor at the initial time of infection, he could have been treated and almost certainly survived. Which of the following describes the appropriate treatment at the time of infection?

A. Antibiotic therapy with a carbapenem and an aminoglycoside

B. Antiviral treatment with cidofovir

C. Immune modulatory therapy with interferon

D. Immune suppression with high-dose steroids and cyclosporine, followed by rituximab

E. Passive immunization with immunoglobulin and active immunization with vaccine

Answers and Explanations

1. Correct: Rabies virus (C)

This is a case of rabies infection caused by the rabies virus, a neurotropic virus of the *Rhabdoviridae* family. It is a negative-sense RNA virus with a characteristic bullet shape appearance in electron microscopy. In the United States, most cases of transmission occur from the bite or scratch of an infected mammal, such as a skunk, bat or raccoon. There are many strains of the virus and they are specific to a particular reservoir host. Transmission by bat bite can actually go unnoticed as they often occur when the patient is asleep and the bat's fangs are small. Transmission due to dog bites and scratches can frequently occur in developing countried that lack animal control and vaccination efforts.

A, B, D, E All of the other answer choices listed do not cause the set of symptoms described in this patient scenario.

2. Correct: Negri bodies (D)

The type of cytopathic effect illustrated in the figure due to rabies infection shows Negri bodies. A Negri body is an eosinophilic inclusion body produced in the cytoplasm of the infected nerve cell. The inclusion body is formed by the synthesis of large quantities of viral proteins and is the site of viral RNA replication. It has been demonstrated that toll-like receptor 3 traffics to the site of viral production and its presence is required for the formation of the Negri body.

A Bielschowsky bodies are associated with Jansky–Bielschowsky disease, a rare genetic disorder of the neuronal ceroid lipofuscinosis (NCL) family of neurodegenerative disorders.

B, C Cowdry bodies are nuclear inclusion bodies with Cowdry type A bodies often associated with infection by herpes simplex virus and varicella-zoster virus, and Cowdry type B bodies often associated with polio and adenovirus infections.

E Paschen bodies are inclusion bodies associated with variola virus infection.

3. Correct: Animal bite (A)

Of the selections offered, the most likely scenario is the bite from an infected animal that resulted in the transmission of saliva to the injury allowing for viral entry into the surrounding musculature and progression to the neuromuscular junction. Rabies virus is transmitted from the saliva of an infected animal and eventually targets human neurons.

B, C, D, E Viral transmission from both a cat litter box as well as sexual transmission would be unable to travel to the central nervous system. Viral entry via an arthropod vector, such as a mosquito bite, could travel to the nervous system; however, rabies virus is not an arthropod-borne pathogen. An unwashed wound is a possible portal of entry of rabies virus; however, the virus is not able to survive in the environment for long periods of time and therefore transmission through a wound is not as likely.

4. Correct: Skin biopsy (E)

The diagnosis of rabies antemortem requires multiple tests. Of the options offered, skin biopsy of hair follicles from the nape of the neck would be the most appropriate. Additional testing of saliva and spinal fluid would also need to be conducted. Antibody testing of serum and cerebrospinal fluid (CSF) would also be done.

A Clinical signs are often non-specific and cannot be used for an antemortem diagnosis.

B Rabies virus is not routinely cultured.

C Western blot is not utilized for diagnostic testing of rabies.

D From this specimen, reverse transcription polymerase chain reaction (RT-PCR) would be required as the molecular test as rabies is an RNA virus (PCR would not be relevant).

5. Correct: Passive immunization with immunoglobulin and active immunization with vaccine (E)

Rabies is a nearly 100% fatal disease once symptoms have appeared. If treated with human rabies immunoglobulin and vaccination at the time or soon after infection, however, the survival is essentially 100%.

A, B, C, D At the time of infection, cidofovir, an antiviral, has no use in the treatment of rabies. Antibiotics, such as carbapenems or aminoglycosides, have no use in a viral infection. Neither immune modulation with interferon nor any form of immune suppression has a role in the treatment of rabies.

Keywords: Encephalitis, rabies, travel, negri bodies

Case 43

Teenager with Headache and Fever

A 19-year-old college sophomore is brought to her physician with a complaint of extreme headache and a high fever. She had been vomiting all day. Upon physical examination, she demonstrated nuchal rigidity and pain with anterior flexion. Purpuric lesions were noted on her lower legs. Laboratory evaluation of the patient's cerebrospinal fluid (CSF) identified 20,000 white blood cells/mL (98% neutrophils, 2% lymphocytes). CSF glucose was 15 mg/dL with a matched serum glucose of 87 mg/dL and protein was 140 mg/dL. A microscopic image of a Gram stain of the CSF is shown in the following figure.

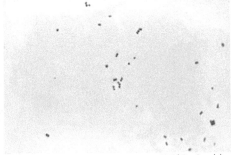

Image courtesy: CDC/ Dr. Brodsky

Questions

1. Which of the following organisms is most likely the cause of this illness?

A. *Haemophilus influenzae*

B. *Neisseria gonorrhoeae*

C. *Neisseria meningitidis*

D. *Moraxella catarrhalis*

E. *Streptococcus pneumonia*

2. Which of the following bacterial products would contribute to the purpuric lesions observed on the patient's legs?

A. Capsule

B. Endotoxin

C. Exotoxin

D. Flagella

E. Immunoglobulin A1 (IgA1) protease

3. Which of the following tests is commonly used to distinguish the causative organism from those of the same genus?

A. Carbohydrate utilization test

B. Catalase test

C. Esculin test

D. Gram stain

E. Quellung reaction

4. There are multiple serogroups that have been identified for this organism. Which of the following is used to determine the serogroup type?

A. Capsule

B. Hyaluronic acid

C. Lipopolysaccharide (LPS)

D. Nucleic acid

E. Pili

5. The patient's boyfriend soon joins her at the hospital, and when he has a chance, he pulls the physician aside and confesses that the two of them had been intimate just 2 days before. The boyfriend asks if he should do anything so that he won't get sick as well. Which of the following best describes what his next step should be?

A. Admission for observation

B. Antibiotics

C. High-dose immunoglobulin

D. No treatment

E. Vaccination

Answers and Explanations

IgA1 protease) do not cause these types of lesions.

1. Correct: *Neisseria meningitidis* (C)

This is a case of bacterial meningitis. While all of the listed organisms can cause meningitis (though rarely with *Neisseria gonorrhoeae* and *Moraxella catarrhalis*), given the scenario, the most likely cause is *Neisseria meningitidis*. A clue to this is the age of the patient as well as the fact that she is a college student. Dormitory living is a risk factor for meningitis from *N. meningitidis* as it is transmitted person-to-person via aerosolization. Additional evidence of *N. meningitidis* is the presence of purpuric lesions on the extremities that can be observed with this infection. Lastly, the Gram stain and microscopy results of this case indicate *N. meningitidis* as the most likely cause, as gram-negative (pink or red) diplococci can be seen in the Gram stain shown in the figure. *N. meningitidis* are aerobic, gram-negative diplococci that can be asymptomatically carried in the nasopharynx of up to 10% of adults. These organisms can be cultured on both blood agar and chocolate agar. Selective media for this organism is Thayer–Martin agar.

A, B, D, E The clinical picture is not compatible with *Haemophilus influenzae*, *N. gonorrhoeae*, *M. catarrhalis*, or *Streptococcus pneumonia*.

2. Correct: Endotoxin (B)

The purpuric or petechial lesions that appear as a result of some bacterial infections is caused by the release of endotoxin into blood. In the case of *N. meningitidis*, the endotoxin is lipo-oligosaccharide (LOS), a shorter version of typical gram-negative LPS. LOS in the blood induces disseminated intravascular coagulation (DIC) that results in insufficient clotting agents being available to prevent these small hemorrhages. These lesions occur in approximately 70% of cases where septicemia has occurred.

A, C, D, E The other virulence factors listed (capsule, exotoxin, flagella, and

3. Correct: Carbohydrate utilization test (A)

Of the tests listed, the carbohydrate utilization test best distinguishes *N. meningitidis* from other pathogenic organisms in the genus *N. gonorrhoeae* or *M. catarrhalis*. *N. meningitidis* utilizes glucose and maltose as the carbon sources in the process of the oxidative Entner–Doudoroff pathway.

B The catalase test is used to distinguish *Staphylococcus* spp. from other gram-positive cocci such as *Streptococcus* spp. and *Enterococcus* spp.

C Esculin test is not used for *N. meningitidis*.

D A Gram stain is only able to distinguish gram-positive and gram-negative organisms from each other and all *Neisseria* spp. have a similar Gram stain morphology.

E Quellung reaction is used for encapsulated organisms such as *Streptococcus pneumoniae*.

4. Correct: Capsule (A)

There are 13 serogroups of *N. meningitidis* identified by the antigenicity of the bacterial capsule polysaccharides. The contribution of each serogroup to the development of disease is associated with age of the patient. Serogroup B predominates in children under the age of 1 year. Serogroups C, Y, and W135 are responsible for the majority of meningococcal disease in individuals over the age of 11 years. Some organisms are typed by pili, but not *N. meningitidis*.

There are two types of vaccines available in the United States for meningococcal disease: conjugate vaccine and serogroup B vaccine. The conjugate vaccines are polyvalent and cover types A, C, W, and Y by conjugating serogroup polysaccharides to diphtheria toxoid. The serogroup B vaccines contain recombinant neisserial proteins from only serogroup B. Vaccination recommendations are in general for children 11 to 12 years of age for the conjugate vaccines and 16 to 23 years of age for the serogroup B vaccines.

B, C These are virulence factors, so these options are not correct.

D This option is incorrect as the genetic sequence of the organism is using for genotyping not serotyping.

E Pili is also a virulence factor.

5. Correct: Antibiotics (B)

Close contacts of patients with *N. meningitidis* include people who live in the same household and anyone who might have had direct contact with the patient's saliva (including boyfriends and girlfriends). All close contacts should receive prophylaxis with appropriate antibiotics. The exact choice of antibiotics is influenced by age and possible resistance in the community but may include ciprofloxacin, ceftriaxone, or rifampin.

A, C, D, E Immunoglobulin has no use in the prevention of *N. meningitidis*. The time for use of vaccination to prevent meningitis is not after exposure, but the vaccine should be administered in early teenage years and before going to college. It would not be appropriate to do nothing or simply observe the boyfriend. Given his degree of contact, it is quite probable that he is also infected but not yet symptomatic. Since this is a potentially deadly disease, prophylaxis is indicated.

Keywords: Meningitis, hemorrhage, *Neisseria meningitidis*, CSF, prophylaxis

Case 44

Elderly Female with Severe Headache and Nausea

A 73-year-old female is seen in the emergency department with symptoms of fever, severe headache, and nausea. She reports that her fever and headache began 2 days ago. Computed tomography (CT) imaging identified inflammation of the meninges. A lumbar puncture is done and an elevated opening pressure is observed. The cerebrospinal fluid (CSF) was sent for laboratory testing and found to have increased number of lymphocytes and polymorphonuclear cells but normal protein levels. A Gram stain of the CSF was negative for bacteria. The CSF was cultured and 2 days later was found to be able to grow at 4°C. A history collected from her daughter reveals that the patient is currently taking treatment for high blood pressure and diabetes. No recent travel is reported. She has a dog and two cats. The patient is generally active and attended a family reunion picnic 3 weeks ago.

Questions

1. Which of the following would most likely be the causative agent of these symptoms?

A. *Cryptococcus neoformans*

B. *Haemophilus influenzae*

C. *Listeria monocytogenes*

D. *Streptococcus agalactiae*

E. West Nile virus

2. Which of the following is most likely the source of this infection?

A. Animal contact

B. Contaminated food

C. Fomite transmission

D. Mosquito bite

E. Person to person

3. Which of the following contributes to cell-to-cell spread?

A. The organism forms syncytia

B. The organism lyses infected cells

C. The organism polymerizes actin

D. The organism is released via exocytosis

E. The organism uses a type IV secretion system

4. In culture, what type of motility is observed with this agent?

A. Gliding

B. Linear

C. Sliding

D. Swarming

E. Tumbling

5. This patient has suspected meningitis. What patient factor would most likely cause the physician to include an additional antibiotic, beyond the standard empirical treatment protocol, to treat the pathogen?

A. Age

B. Diabetes

C. Duration of symptoms

D. Elevated opening pressure

E. Having pets

Answers and Explanations

The symptoms presented in this scenario are indicative of meningitis as described in the CT findings. All of the agents offered are capable of causing meningitis, but given the patient's age, the first consideration would be for either *Streptococcus pneumoniae* or *Listeria monocytogenes*. The CSF profile identified a preponderance of lymphocytes that could indicate a viral etiology. This would also be supported by the lack of microscopic detection of bacteria. However, the ability to culture the organism at 4°C would identify *Listeria* spp. as the cause as *Listeria* spp. can grow between 1 and 45°C. *L. monocytogenes* are gram-positive bacilli, but they might not be microscopically detected in CSF due to few organisms being present. However, the organisms would become visible upon culture. A Gram stain of the culture would look similar to the following microscopic image.

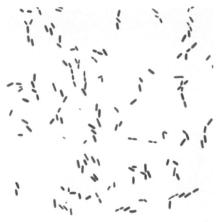

Image courtesy: Lisa D'Angelo

A, B, D, E None of the other agents listed can grow at this lower temperature. The fact that the organism grew on culture excludes West Nile virus.

2. Correct: Contaminated food (B)
The patient history provided by the woman's daughter identifies a family picnic in the recent past. This scenario also supports the diagnosis of *L. monocytogenes* as contaminated food is often the source of infection. While gastroenteritis caused by *L. monocytogenes* usually manifests within 24 hours of exposure, invasive disease can occur up to 28 days postexposure.

A, C, D, E *L. monocytogenes* is not commonly transmitted by any of the other methods listed. *Listeria* spp. is not an arthropod-borne infection nor is there an animal reservoir.

3. Correct: The organism polymerizes actin (C)

Listeria spp. is a facultative intracellular bacterium that can infect cells via the activity of internalins. Internalins are one of several virulence factors utilized by the bacteria to gain entry into cells. These proteins are located on the surface of the bacteria and are thought to result in the interaction with host cell receptors E-cadherin and Met. This interaction results in the adhesion of the bacteria to the cell and the induction of phagocytosis. By this mechanism, *Listeria* spp. can enter the cell and evade the host immune response. The bacterium lyses the phagocytic vacuole by activity of the pore-forming toxin listeriolysin O and is released in the cell cytoplasm. Once in the cell, *Listeria* spp. polymerizes actin filaments to propel itself through the cytoplasm utilizing the actin polymerization machinery usurped by the bacterial protein Act A. This movement through the cytoplasm can project the bacteria from one cell into the next to result in bacterial spread.
A The organism does not induce syncytia formation in infected cells.
B The organism does not lyse the infected cell but does lyse the phagocytic vacuole.
D The organism is not released outside of the infected cell via an exocytosis mechanism.
E A type IV secretion system is used to transport macromolecules across a cell membrane. It is not involved in the release of organisms from an infected cell.

4. Correct: Tumbling (E)

Bacterial motility occurs in a variety of manners and occurs for a variety of reasons, including chemotaxis. *Listeria* spp., in culture, has a characteristic motility known as tumbling motility. Tumbling occurs due to multiple peritrichous flagella present around the bacillus. Tumbling occurs at temperatures other than 37°C. At this temperature, the bacteria reduce the flagellar activity and utilize the actin propulsion mechanism as a means of moving within the host cell. *Listeria* spp. motility appears to be important for biofilm formation. Biofilms allow for bacterial attachment to surfaces and may be important for foodborne transmission. One assay to detect *Listeria* spp. is the motility test where cultures are grown at 18 to 25°C in semisolid motility medium. The organism is inoculated by stab method and umbrella-shaped growth away from the stab entry point is indicative of *L. monocytogenes*. Additionally, tumbling motility can be observed microscopically.

A, B, C, D These options are incorrect as these other forms of motility are not observed with *Listeria*.

5. Correct: Age (A)

The empiric treatment of suspected meningitis is well established and consists of ceftriaxone and vancomycin (unless contraindicated due to a patient factor such as allergy) to cover the most common organisms involved (*Streptococcus pneumoniae*, group *B. Streptococcus, Haemophilus influenzae*, and *Neisseria meningtides*). When a patient is younger than 1 month or older than 50 years old , they are also at higher risk for *L. monocytogenes* meningitis, and ampicillin should be added to the regimen empirically.

B, C, D, E None of the other factors listed without additional specific information would change the empiric antibiotic regimen.

Keywords: Listeria, intracellular, virulence factors, meningitis, tumbling motility

Case 45

Adult Female with Headache and Disorientation

A 64-year-old female is brought to the emergency department in September by her husband who is concerned that she is disoriented. He states that she has been experiencing headache and body aches for the past week. Upon physical examination, she displays signs of nuchal rigidity and lower extremity weakness. Her vital signs are a temperature of 38.8°C, blood pressure of 130/77 mmHg, and heart rate of 84 bpm. Past medical history indicates that the patient is currently being treated for hypertension. The patient's husband reports that they had attended a Labor Day picnic the week previous and oddly he noticed that there was a cleanup crew in the park taking away several dead birds. A lumbar puncture was performed and analysis of the cerebrospinal fluid (CSF) identified a white blood cell (WBC) count of 228 cells/mm^3, with a preponderance of lymphocytes. Protein was 100 mg/dL and glucose was normal.

Questions

1. Which of the following organisms is most likely responsible for this patient's symptoms?

A. Herpes simplex virus (HSV)

B. West Nile virus (WNV)

C. *Neisseria meningitidis*

D. *Haemophilus influenzae*

E. Epstein–Barr Virus (EBV)

2. What is the greatest risk factor for increased mortality due to this disease?

A. Activity

B. Age

C. Gender

D. Hypertension

E. Diabetes

3. Which of the following is the primary host for the most likely causative agent?

A. Birds

B. Humans

C. Mosquitoes

D. Rodents

E. Horses

4. Which of the following would be the most common evidence to confirm this patient's infection?

A. Acute immunoglobulin M (IgM) to convalescent IgM titers

B. Culture

C. Point-of-care rapid antibody test

D. Reverse transcriptase polymerase chain reaction (RT-PCR)

E. Serology for IgM, IgG, and IgA

5. Which of the following would be the most appropriate treatment for this patient's infection?

A. Ceftriaxone

B. Acyclovir

C. Intravenous immunoglobulin (IVIg)

D. Brincidofovir

E. Supportive care only

Answers and Explanations

1. Correct: West Nile virus (WNV) (B)

The description of this patient's symptoms with disorientation and muscle weakness suggests encephalitis. The CSF findings describe a viral infection where usually lymphocytes predominate and protein levels are high. The brief history given of this patient implicates a Labor Day picnic as a predecessor to her symptoms. As WNV is transmitted by mosquito bite, the most likely transmission scenario is infection during the picnic. Furthermore, the timing in early September (Labor Day) is at the peak of West Nile prevalence (WNV typically appears in mid-July through early October), and the noted dead birds likely indicate the virus killing the primary host. The figure below shows an electron micrograph of WNV particles.

A HSV could produce encephalitis and should be considered in a differential. However, the facts of the case point to West Nile virus as the causative agent.

C, D These are bacterial causes of meningitis. Risk factors for *Neisseria* include contact with infected individuals in an institutional setting. Infection with *Haemophilus* is less likely due to the availability of routine vaccination.

E EBV too could produce encephalitis and should be considered in a differential. However, the facts of the case point to West Nile virus as the most likely causative agent.

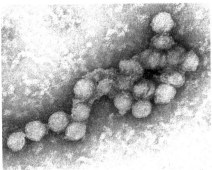

Image courtesy: CDC/ P.E. Rollin

2. Correct: Age (B)

The risk of severe symptoms increases for patients over the age of 60 (such as the patient described in this case). Additionally, individuals with certain underlying chronic diseases and transplant recipients are also at increased risk.

A, C, D, E Activity, gender, diabetes, and hypertension are not known risk factors for WNV infection.

3. Correct: Birds (A)

When WNV first came to the United States in 1999, it was noted that birds were the primary host of the virus. In particular, song birds had high viral titers. Several avian species were utilized as sentinels to monitor the spread of the virus during the epidemiological investigations.

B, C, D, E The *Culex* species of mosquito is the vector for the virus (see figure below), biting first the infected host bird and then the human recipients. Although humans are infected by the virus, human-to-human spread is not likely as virus does not reach very high titers in mammals and viremia is short-lived. As such, mammals are considered to be dead-end hosts for this virus.

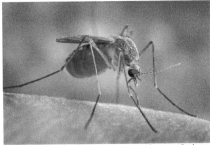

Image courtesy: CDC/ James Gathany

4. Correct: Acute immunoglobulin M (IgM) to convalescent IgM titers (A)

If symptoms and patient history suggest WNV, the most common test to confirm infection is enzyme-linked immunosorbent assay (ELISA) for comparison of acute IgM antibody titers to convalescent IgM antibody titers. Currently, there are four commercial ELISA antibody tests that are approved by the Food and Drug Administration (FDA). These have a specificity of 92 to 98% and sensitivity of 96 to 100%.

B, C, D, E Viral culture and molecular testing to detect viral nucleic acids can be used to confirm an infection but are used less frequently mostly because viremia peaks around the time of symptoms, and the ability to detect WNV after initial seroconversion quickly decreases. At present, there are no point-of-care rapid tests approved for WNV detection.

5. Correct: Supportive care only (E)

As with many viral infections, the treatment for WNV infection is supportive care. **A, B, C, D** While many antivirals have been tried, none has shown particular success against the infection. Appropriate controlled studies are not available at present. Of particular note, IVIg from areas where WNV was endemic was considered and case reports can be found suggesting its benefit. However, there is no evidence from clinical trials that show a benefit for this form of treatment.

Keywords: Encephalitis, West Nile virus, arbovirus, serology

Case 46

Adult Male with Headache for Several Months

A 50-year-old male comes to the emergency room complaining of a headache which has persisted for several months. He has been to his primary care physician (PCP), several urgent care clinics, and even two other emergency rooms. He is generally in good health and takes no medications. He reports that he smokes a quarter pack of cigarettes a day for the past 30 years. He has no recent travel, no unusual exposures to animals, and no sick contacts. He does not drink alcohol and does not use any illicit drugs. He is single and sexually active with multiple partners but has had routine testing for HIV and other sexually transmitted infections (STIs) through the department of health, and his last tests were all negative. His most recent negative testing for HIV and other STIs was 1 month prior to the onset of symptoms, and he states he had not had any sexual contacts since at least 1 month prior to that. A review of the patient's medical records reveals that both his PCP and one urgent care center thought the headache was sinusitis, and the other urgent care center thought it was tension headaches. The emergency rooms dismissed him as drug seeking.

Because of the chronicity and lack of improvement, a computed tomography (CT) of the head was ordered and was negative. A lumbar puncture (LP) was then performed. Opening pressure from the LP in left lateral decubitus position was 250 mm H_2O, protein was 80 mg/dL, glucose was 5 mg/dL with a corresponding serum glucose of 100, the white blood cell (WBC) count in the cerebrospinal fluid (CSF) was 200 cells/mm^3 with 75% monocytes. A stain of the CSF reveals the organisms seen in the figure below.

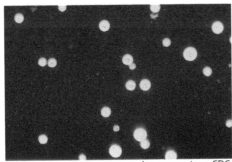

Image courtesy: CDC

Questions

1. Which of the following pathogens is the most likely cause of this patient's symptoms?

A. *Candida albicans*

B. *Cryptococcus neoformans*

C. *Neisseria meningitides*

D. *Staphylococcus aureus*

E. *Streptococcus pneumonia*

2. What is the most likely stain used to visualize the causative organism in the figure?

A. Acridine orange

B. Brown and Brenn

C. Gentian violet

D. Gram stain

E. India ink

3. A strain deficient in producing which of the following structures would have lower pathogenicity and decreased or absent staining?

A. Capsule

B. Cell wall

C. Envelope

D. Golgi apparatus

E. Inner membrane

4. Which of the following enzymes is an important virulence factor for the causative organism?

A. Hyaluronidase

B. Phenol oxidase

C. Polyphosphate kinase

D. RNAse B

E. Urease

5. Which of the following is the most appropriate initial therapy for this patient?

A. Albendazole

B. Amphotericin B and flucytosine

C. Ceftriaxone and vancomycin

D. Fluconazole

E. Meropenem

Answers and Explanations

1. Correct: *Cryptococcus neoformans* (B)

What is described in this case are the classic signs and symptoms of cryptococcal meningitis in a nonimmunosuppressed individual. The causative agent is the yeast *Cryptococcus neoformans*. While HIV and other immunodeficient states, such as solid organ transplant, are the typical risk factors for developing cryptococcal meningitis, approximately 30% of cryptococcal meningitis in HIV-negative patients occurs in patients with no apparent immune issues. The classic findings are an unrelenting headache, sometime associated with fever, with no apparent cause. Because of the subacute nature of this infection, patients often go from doctor to doctor until a diagnosis is finally made. The diagnostic clues in this case are the high opening pressure, the extremely low glucose, the mononuclear pleocytosis seen in the CSF, and the causative organism shown microscopically in the figure, which is *C. neoformans*.

A, C, D, E *Candida albicans* is not a typical cause of meningitis. The large round yeast form also excludes the bacteria listed as answer choices: *Neisseria meningitides* (gram-negative), *Staphylococcus aureus* (gram-positive), and *Streptococcus pneumonia* (gram-positive).

2. Correct: India ink (E)

The classic stain for *C. neoformans* is India ink which stains the yeast form and the background but shows negative staining of the capsule and gives the halo effect seen in the figure. Currently, the cryptococcal antigen test, where capsular polysaccharide antigens are detected by latex agglutination or enzyme immunoassay, is more commonly used in clinical microbiology laboratories.

A Acridine orange is a fluorescent dye which binds nucleic acids and is used to stain phagosome contents.

B, C Brown and Brenn is a Gram stain of tissue and gentian violet is a component of the Gram stain.

D Gram stain is used for typical bacteria, but some fungi can also be visualized by Gram stain; however, *C. neoformans* stains poorly with Gram stain because of the large capsule.

3. Correct: Capsule (A)

Because the causative agent, *C. neoformans*, is most easily viewed microscopically when the thick capsule is a negative halo stained with India ink, capsule-deficient strains would not be visualized using this negative stain. The polysaccharide capsule also allows *Cryptococcus* spp. to evade the immune system by preventing phagocytosis. Strains which are deficient in the capsule undergo increased phagocytosis and are therefore less virulent.

B While *C. neoformans* does possess a cell wall, this component is not responsible for the evasion of the immune system.

C Envelope is a component of viruses derived from the host cell such as in Herpes Simplex virus.

D, E These are components of the human host cell.

4. Correct: Phenol oxidase (B)

The fungal enzyme phenol oxidase is a key component of the metabolic pathway that synthesizes melanin, which is a virulence factor in *Cryptococcus* spp. Strains that produce melanin are less susceptible to phagocytosis and oxidative damage.

A Hyaluronidase is produced by *S. pyogenes* and is an important virulence factor in skin infections.

C Polyphosphate kinase catalyzes the formation of adenosine triphosphate (ATP) and is not considered to be a virulence factor.

D *C. neoformans* does not produce RNAse B

E Urease is an enzyme that is a virulence factor for some gastrointestinal pathogens such as *Helicobacter pylori*. Although many strains of *C. neoformans* do produce urease, it is not considered an important virulence factor of this pathogen.

5. Correct: Amphotericin B and flucytosine (B)

Treatment of cryptococcosis is complex, but the initial treatment is an induction phase generally with a combination of liposomal amphotericin B and flucytosine. This combination has been shown to be the most rapidly fungicidal and has improved mortality over amphotericin B alone or amphotericin B in combination with fluconazole.

A Albendazole is an antihelminthic used for the treatment of various parasitic worms.

C Ceftriaxone and vancomycin would be used for empiric treatment of suspected bacterial meningitis.

D Fluconazole is used in the consolidation phase of the treatment of cryptococcal meningitis but is not generally used as the initial treatment.

E Meropenem can often be substituted for ceftriaxone in patients with a penicillin allergy due to high penetration to the CSF and low cross-allergenicity with other beta-lactams; however, it has no use in treating *Cryptococcus.*

Keywords: *Cryptococcus neoformans*, fungal meningitis, capsule, India ink, phenol oxidase, amphotericin B, flucytosine

Case 47

Febrile Teenager with Headache and Neck Stiffness

A 17-year-old male is seen in the emergency department (ED) with a 24-hour history of severe headache, vomiting, neck rigidity, and fever. Patient history included a recent spring break camping trip to South Carolina that included a river rafting excursion. Physical examination reveals a temperature of 103°F, a blood pressure of 127/88 mmHg, and a heart rate of 121 bpm. A magnetic resonance imaging (MRI) shows basal meningeal enhancement. A lumbar puncture was performed, and analysis of the cerebrospinal fluid (CSF) showed signs of hemorrhage with glucose less than 20 mg/dL, protein level of 469 mg/dL, and neutrophilic pleocytosis with a white cell count of 8,250 cells/mm^3. A wet mount of the CSF revealed bodies represented in the following figure. A Giemsa stain revealed similar results (data not shown). The patient was started on multiple antibiotics, antivirals, and antifungals as well as steroids; however, 2 days after presentation to the ED, the patient became comatose and he died 3 days after admission.

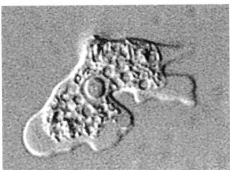

Image courtesy: CDC

Questions

1. Which of the following is most likely the cause of this patient's condition?

A. *Histoplasma capsulatum*

B. Herpes simplex virus (HSV)

C. *Naegleria fowleri*

D. Rabies virus

E. *Taenia solium*

2. How did this patient most likely acquire this infection?

A. Exposure to contaminated soil

B. Exposure to contaminated water

C. Exposure to contaminated food

D. Being bitten by mosquitos

E. Being bitten by a rodent

3. Which of the following best describes the infectious form of the causative pathogen?

A. Cyst stage

B. Flagellated stage

C. Larval stage

D. Trophozoite stage

E. Endospore stage

4. Which of the following is most likely the patient's route of exposure to the causative organism?

A. Intradermal exposure

B. Pulmonary exposure

C. Gastric exposure

D. Intranasal exposure

E. Direct inoculation of the CSF

5. Patients with this disease often have which of the following conditions that predispose them to the infection?

A. An anatomic defect allowing the organism to pass the blood–brain barrier

B. A defect in the neuronal sheaths allowing direct infection of neuronal tissue

C. A hypersensitivity to the toxin produced by the organism

D. A specific, and often, undiagnosed defect in natural killer cells

E. No condition has been identified that increases risk of this infection

Answers and Explanations

1. Correct: *Naegleria fowleri* (C)

This is a case of primary amoebic meningoencephalitis (PAM). PAM is a brain pathology resulting from the digestion of neural cells by the parasite *N. fowleri*. Diagnosis of this organism is most often by microscopy and polymerase chain reaction (PCR). The symptoms are those of meningitis and include blood in the CSF resulting from hemorrhagic activity. There is a very high mortality with this infection due to its rapid progression. Fortunately, infection is rare. As of the year 2017, there have only been 142 cases in the United States since 1962 with a 95% fatality rate. Lack of response to multiple forms of treatment is a clue that the organism is not one that responds to standard therapies; however this does not exclude many of the choices listed for this question. The image of the amoeba shown above makes *Naegleria fowleri* the clear causative agent of this patient's infection.
A *Histoplasma capsulatum* is a fungus that has more of an appearance of a knobby sphere.
B, D These are viruses that would not be visualized on a wet mount slide or by Giemsa stain.
E *Taenia solium* is a tapeworm and the morphologies identified would be proglottids or worm eggs.

2. Correct: Exposure to contaminated water (B)

This parasite resides in natural warm fresh water pools in general but has been detected in poorly chlorinated swimming pools as well. It is able to withstand temperatures of approximately 115°F but does not tend to grow in cooler waters. Thus, it is much more commonly seen in the southern United States and not typically in the north.
A, C, D, E Contaminated soil and food are incorrect choices, and there is no evidence of an arthropod vector or animal host for this infection.

3. Correct: Trophozoite stage (D)

The infectious form of *N. fowleri* is the trophozoite. This is the stage of the parasite that is capable of feeding and causing PAM.
A The cyst stage of the pathogen is able to evade the immune system of the host and forms a protective coat similar to a bacterial spore when the environment becomes harsh. Cysts can also be inhaled, but the trophozoite is the disease-causing stage.
B Trophozoites are able to become flagellated and motile temporarily. These motile forms are also not capable of causing disease but can be a means of microscopic identification.
C, E There is no larval or endospore stage in *N. fowleri*.

4. Correct: Intranasal exposure (D)

Infection by *Naegleria* species occurs when contaminated water gets up the nose and is deeply inhaled. There are no other major transmission mechanisms. Swimming in contaminated water has been identified as the source of many infections, but transmission by neti pots has also been documented. The parasite is thought to pass through the nasal mucosa and enters the brain via the olfactory neuroepithelia. Why there are so few infections is not known and may be a result of host–pathogen interactions, with some individuals being more susceptible to PAM.
A, B, C, E This parasite enters the brain via the nasal mucosa and olfactory neuroepithelia. Intradermal, pulmonary or gastric exposure is not a method of gaining access to the brain. Direct inoculation of the CSF could only occur if there was damage to the skull or spinal cord.

5. Correct: No condition has been identified that increases risk of this infection (E)

PAM is a rare condition, and in most cases, there is no specific issue identified that puts patients at increased risk of infection. Exposure to the pathogen seems much more common than infection, based on serologic studies. This implies that those who do become infected may have some subtle deficit, or it may simply be that exposure via other routes, such as ingestion, causes an immune response without a risk for encephalitis.

A, B, C, D Each of these hypotheses has been posited but there is currently no evidence to support one mechanism over another for all reported cases.

Keywords: *Naegleria fowleri*, meninigoencephalitis, parasite

Case 48

Travelers with Acute Febrile Illness

A heterosexual couple returned from their 10-year anniversary vacation after spending a week in Punta Cana in the Dominican Republic. While there, they spent time at a resort and had an overnight trip into the rain forest. They ate native foods and drank water from the tap on the overnight trip.

About a week after returning to the United States, both experienced high fevers, chills, headaches, sweats, and fatigue. They both thought they had a virus, but the symptoms worsened and the fevers were noted to be as high as 40°C. The wife called 911 a week later and they both were taken to the hospital. Upon questioning, the couple indicated that they did not utilize a travel clinic prior to their trip and took no medication or vaccinations. They did not use insect repellent or mosquito netting regularly.

Shortly after admission to the hospital, the 41-year-old husband developed seizures. On examination, he appeared postictal, pale, sweaty, and was breathing rapidly. His vitals were heart rate (HR) 120 bpm, respiratory rate (RR) 30 breaths/min, temperature 39°C, and blood pressure (BP) 90/60 mmHg. His sclerae were noted to be icteric. The remainder of his examination was essentially normal.

On examination, the 40-year-old wife appeared anxious but was otherwise in no distress. Her vitals were HR 90 bpm, RR 20 breaths/min, temperature 38.3°C, and BP 122/78 mm Hg. It was noted that she had an enlarged spleen.

Blood cultures, a complete blood count (CBC), and a chem 20 were drawn for both patients, and at the suggestion of an infectious diseases consultation, blood smears and serological testing for dengue, yellow fever, Zika, hepatitis A, B, and C, and chikungunya were sent but will take some time to come back with results. Urine was also collected and the husband's urine was dark and tea-colored.

The CBC and chem 20 showed the following relevant tests.

	Husband	Wife
WBC	3.2	5.4
Hemoglobin	6.8	8.8
Platelet	75	110
Aspartate aminotransferase (AST)	48	32
Alanine aminotransferase (ALT)	52	27
TB	2.5	1.0
DB	0.5	0.5

Questions

1. These patients were infected through which of the following intervening agents?

A. *Aedes aegypti*

B. *Anopheles gambiae*

C. Contaminated food

D. Contaminated water

E. Direct person-to-person spread

2. Based on the blood smear shown in the figure below which of the following pathogens is the most likely cause of the infection?

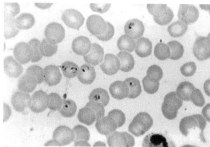

Image courtesy: CDC/ Steven Glenn, Laboratory & Consultation Division

A. *Babesia microti*

B. Chikungunya virus

C. Dengue virus

D. Hepatitis A virus

E. *Plasmodium falciparum*

3. Which of the following life cycle forms can be seen in the above figure?

A. Amastigote

B. Cyst

C. Maltese cross

D. Schizont

E. Trophozoite

4. Which of the following cell types does this organism first infect upon entry into the body?

A. Hepatocyte

B. Megakaryocyte

C. Splenocyte

D. Red blood cell

E. White blood cell

5. The husband has another witnessed seizure, so he is transferred to the intensive care unit (ICU) for monitoring. Which of the following treatments would be the most appropriate to initiate for the husband at this time?

A. Vancomycin and piperacillin–tazobactam

B. Hepatitis A hyperimmune immunoglobulin G (IgG)

C. Chloroquine

D. Quinidine gluconate and doxycycline

E. Supportive care and antiseizure medications

Answers and Explanations

1. Correct: *Anopheles gambiae* (B)

This is a case of malaria, caused by *Plasmodium falciparum*. See the explanation for Question 2 for more information explaining why *P. falciparum* is the most likely causative agent. Malaria is transmitted by the *Anopheles gambiae* mosquito. The patients in this case mentioned that they did not receive any pretravel medication or vaccinations, so they therefore were not protected with prophylaxis medication to protect against malaria. They also did not use insect repellent or mosquito netting regularly during their trip, so they did not actively prevent mosquito bites or transmission of the parasite. As a result, these two patients were at risk for malaria while in this endemic area of the world.

A, C, D, E Though they were exposed, *P. falciparum* is not transmitted by contaminated food, water, or by person-to-person contact. *Aedes aegypti* is also a mosquito vector, but these mosquitoes are responsible for transmission of the viruses of yellow fever, dengue, chikungunya, and Zika.

2. Correct: *Plasmodium falciparum* (E)

This is a case of malaria, caused by *P. falciparum*. A most recognized form of the *Plasmodium* spp. parasite is the ring form observed in infected red blood cells (seen in the figure). The ring form is distinctive for *P. falciparum* species. The viral genotypes listed would not be identifiable in a microscopic evaluation of a blood smear. The wife likely has uncomplicated malaria, but the husband has severe malaria and almost certainly cerebral malaria, one of the deadliest forms with a 20% mortality even with rapid and appropriate treatment. There are several diseases that can cause the described illnesses and are associated with travel to the Dominican Republic.

The most common would be malaria but also common could be dengue virus and chikungunya virus.

A, B, C, D Hepatitis A is frequently seen in travelers as well, but the symptoms described in these two patients are not typical for hepatitis and the changes in the liver function tests (LFTs) are too mild to indicate hepatitis A. The high spiking fevers seen are a classic sign to indicate malaria. *Babesia* spp. infections also have findings on blood smear, but this is typically a Maltese cross, and *Babesia* spp. infections are not typically found in the Dominican Republic. All malaria in the Dominican Republic is *P. falciparum*, and it is one of the few places which still has chloroquine-sensitive malaria infections. This couple should have seen a travel clinic before their trip and taken precautions to prevent this infection. This illness could have been prevented with appropriate prophylaxis.

3. Correct: Trophozoite (E)

The ring form of *P. falciparum* is the trophozoite stage of the parasitic life cycle, seen in the figure.

A, B, C, D The other stages are the schizont and merozoite. The amastigote is a stage in the life cycle of *Leishmania*. The cyst form is observed in other parasites such as *Naegleria fowleri*. The Maltese cross is the term used to describe *Babesia* spp. merozoites.

4. Correct: Hepatocyte (A)

Malarial disease results in the lysis of red blood cells causing an anemic condition. This is an end-stage effect of the parasitic life cycle. The cycle begins with the bite of an infected mosquito. During the taking of a blood meal the parasite sporozoites are transmitted to the person. The first cells to be infected by the parasite are hepatocytes. These mature to form tissue schizonts that contain merozoites. The schizonts rupture and the merozoites are released into the bloodstream and then go on to infect red blood cells.

The lysis of the red cells occurs due to a several activities of the parasite within the cell. First the red blood cell hemoglobin is digested leaving a toxic metabolite termed hemozoin as the merozoite matures to the trophozoite and then matures schizont stages. The parasite also reduces membrane deformability preventing the cell to appropriately respond to applied stress.

B Megkaryocytes are bone marrow progenitor cells having a large nucleus. They are not known to be infected in the life cycle of *Plasmodium* spp.

C Splenocytes are white blood cells residing in the spleen.

D Red blood cells are a target of the parasite but not the first cell that becomes infected post transmission.

E White blood cells are not infected by the parasite.

5. Correct: Quinidine gluconate and doxycycline (D)

The treatment for severe malaria (no matter what region of the world that the patient was infected in) is currently quinidine gluconate plus one of the following drugs: doxycycline, tetracycline, or clindamycin. In the case described here, the appropriate choice is quinidine plus doxycycline. The treatment should be given parenterally, and the quinidine should have a loading dose to reach appropriate levels rapidly. Artesunate can be considered instead of quinidine but is considered investigational and only available from the Centers for Disease Control and Prevention (CDC) in the United States.

A, B Vancomycin, piperacillin–tazobactam, and hepatitis A IgG have no use in treating malaria.

C Chloroquine alone would not be sufficient to treat severe malaria.

E In a patient with these severe symptoms, supportive care alone would not suffice.

Keywords: Malaria, blood, *Plasmodium falciparum*, quinidine gluconate, *Anopheles* spp. mosquito

Case 49

Newborn with Jaundice

A 27-year-old mother of a 4-year old boy was expecting her second child. At 35 weeks' gestation, a girl was delivered by emergency cesarean section due to preeclampsia. Routine group *B. Streptococcus* (GBS) testing of the mother was negative. The neonate was 16.1 inches and 3.9 pounds at birth (both below the second percentile). Upon physical examination, the baby appeared to be jaundiced with elevated alanine aminotransferase and bilirubin levels. Petechiae were seen on the baby's face and trunk and hepatosplenomegaly was also noted. The mother did not have any additional medical issues at the time of delivery. However, the mother did report having a flu-like illness at 13 weeks of gestation (during the first trimester) that resolved spontaneously. She had not mentioned that illness to her obstetrician at that time because it seemed minor. At that time, several children at her son's day care had typical illnesses, such as upper respiratory infections and enteroviruses. Blood cultures from the newborn were negative.

Questions

1. Which of the following pathogens most likely contributed to this baby's condition?

A. Cytomegalovirus (CMV)

B. Herpes simplex virus (HSV)

C. Lymphocytic choriomeningitis virus

D. Rubella

E. *Streptococcus agalactiae*

2. What is the most common consequence for the mother as a result of this infection?

A. Cardiac issue

B. Hearing loss

C. Neurological deficit

D. No serious consequence

E. Pneumonia

3. For which of the following long-term health problems is this baby most at risk from this infection?

A. Hearing loss

B. Joint stiffness

C. Rash

D. Sterility

E. Septicemia

4. What is the best means to confirm infection in this child?

A. Clinical sign and symptoms

B. Immunoglobulin G (IgG) enzyme-linked immunosorbent assay (ELISA) in mother

C. IgM ELISA in infant

D. Quantitative polymerase chain reaction (PCR) 3 weeks post birth

E. Viral culture of infant saliva

5. The suspected diagnosis is confirmed. What is the most appropriate therapy for the infant to prevent progression of the disease and improve the outcome?

A. No treatment, the damage is not reversible

B. Acyclovir

C. Ganciclovir

D. Cidofovir

E. Penicillin

Answers and Explanations

1. Correct: Cytomegalovirus (CMV) (A)

This is a case of CMV infection in a neo-natal patient following a primary infection of the mother with CMV infection. CMV is one of the TORCH infections which convey significant risk to neonates either congenitally or perinatally. The TORCH infections include Toxoplasmosis, Other (syphilis, varicella-zoster virus [VZV], and parvovirus B19 are the most common), Rubella, CMV, and HSV. It is likely that the mother was infected due to exposure at her son's day care. Day care workers and those who are in close contact with young children are at increased risk for infection by CMV. The most common timing of intrauterine transmission is during the first trimester (as seen in this case). According to the Centers for Disease Control and Prevention (CDC), nearly half of all women are infected prior to pregnancy. It is believed that 50 to 75% of congenital CMV infections are due to reinfection or reactivation in mothers by the virus. All of the pathogens listed in this question should be considered in the differential for the infection described.

B HSV infection is less likely in this case, given the mother has not reported any HSV risk nor were blisters noted. However, HSV often goes underreported by mothers and should be ruled out to confirm the diagnosis. What makes HSV less likely is that the majority of the cases of neonatal HSV are transmitted during vaginal delivery either in a symptomatic or asymptomatic mother with HSV-2 infection. This child was delivered by cesarean section which greatly reduces the risk of HSV.

C, D, E The other options listed (lymphocytic choriomeningitis virus, rubella virus, and *Streptococcus agalactiae*) do not commonly present as described in this case. Furthermore, *S. agalactiae* would normally be identified in the GBS testing as *S. agalactiae* is also known as GBS.

2. Correct: No serious consequence (D)

There are usually no consequences to the mother's infection unless there is a severe immunocompromised state (which is not true of this particular case). However, the consequences listed can all be observed in infected neonates and are therefore potentially very serious.

A, B, C, E The other options are incorrect for this particular case.

3. Correct: Hearing loss (A)

CMV can become a serious infection in those individuals who are immunocompromised. Infants who are premature and of very low birth weight as well as congenitally infected are also at serious risk of CMV infection. Babies who have signs of CMV at birth (including low birth weight, lung, liver, and spleen problems or seizures) are at increased risk for long-term health problems such as vision and hearing loss, mental retardation, seizures, and lack of muscle control. Sensorineural hearing loss is the most common sequela of congenital CMV and is as high as 50%. It is often delayed in onset and can be subtle, and frequently progressive. Infection can lead to profound hearing loss as the child ages.

B, C Joint stiffness and rash are symptoms of CMV infection apparent at birth but are not long-term sequelae.

D Sterility is not reported as a long-term manifestation of congenital CMV infection.

E Septicemia is blood poisoning due to bacteria or their toxins. CMV is a virus.

4. Correct: Viral culture of infant saliva (E)

The best test for the diagnosis of congenital infection is detection of virus in the amniotic fluid by PCR or culture prior to birth if CMV is suspected. Cell culture of CMV is the traditional method of detection utilizing human fibroblast cells. Viral infection results in distinctive cytopathic effects described as owl' eye inclusion bodies as exemplified in the first figure below. A modified culture method using fibroblasts cultured on cover slips is also available.

Virus is then detected by monoclonal fluorescent antibody directed against immediate early viral antigens as shown in the second figure.

Postpartum diagnosis of the infant should be conducted within 3 weeks of birth to confirm congenital infection versus postnatal infection.

A CMV is not diagnosed by clinical signs and symptoms alone.

B, C CMV should not be diagnosed based on detected antibody from either the mother or the child. CMV reactivity of the mother, especially as IgM can be detectable upon reinfection in the mother or persist for several months after the initial infection. Being newly born, serology may be less reliable for CMV infection diagnosis in the child, with antibodies being transferred from the mother.

D PCR can be used to determine infection in the new born but should be done within three weeks of birth to rule out infection acquired during or after delivery.

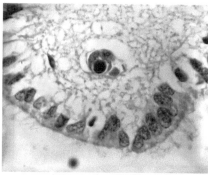

Image courtesy: CDC/ Rosalie B. Haraszti

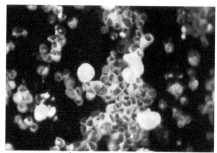

Image courtesy: CDC/ Dr. Craig Lyerla

5.   Correct: Ganciclovir (C)

The most effective antiviral for CMV in general is ganciclovir. Use of ganciclovir is warranted in this case, at least 6 months after the child was likely infected in utero.

A Multiple clinical trials have shown significant improvement in children treated with ganciclovir or valganciclovir as comparted to placebo.

B, D Acyclovir has less activity, and cidofovir is reserved for cases of ganciclovir resistance due to significant toxicities.

E Penicillin would be used to treat GBS or *S. agalactiae* but has no role in the treatment of CMV.

Keywords: Congenital infection, neonate, CMV, TORCH infections, ganciclovir

Case 50

Teenager with Pain in Groin

A 13-year-old boy is brought to the emergency room of a rural hospital by his parents in the summer with a fever and a pain in his groin area. The family lives on a nearby horse ranch in rural Northern New Mexico. The boy was sent home early that morning from a nearby outdoor summer sleepaway camp with a headache, chills, and a fever. The parents say that he complained of sharp pain in his upper legs a few hours later. When questioned more about the camp, the patient mentions that when he was playing in the woods with his friends 5 days earlier, they found some dead mice in a nest. He has also been canoeing and swimming in a local pond throughout his time at camp. Physical examination reveals an ill-appearing boy with a temperature of 103.6°F, blood pressure (BP) of 110/70, and pulse of 115 bpm. There is pain and significant swelling of the left inguinal lymph node and it appears to be fluctuant. The remainder of his examination is unremarkable. Blood is drawn for routine testing. White blood cell (WBC) count is 20,000/µL, and thrombocytopenia is present. Aspiration from the swollen lymph node was collected and sent for Gram stain and culture. A Gram stain is shown in the following figure.

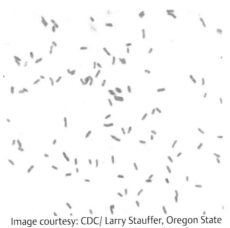

Image courtesy: CDC/ Larry Stauffer, Oregon State
Public Health Laboratory

Questions

1. Which of the following organisms is the most likely causative agent?

A. *Bacillus anthracis*

B. *Borrelia burgdorferi*

C. *Coxiella burnetii*

D. *Francisella tularensis*

E. *Yersinia pestis*

2. Which of the following is the most likely source of this patient's infection?

A. Another camper

B. Horses

C. Mosquitoes

D. Mice

E. Pond

3. Which of the following is an important virulence factor of the most likely causative agent?

A. Exotoxin A

B. Lipopolysaccharide (LPS)

C. Lipoteichoic acid

D. Pili

E. Urease

4. The causative agent of this patient's symptoms is listed as a category A bioterrorism agent by the Centers for Disease Control and Prevention (CDC). Which of the following microorganisms is also a category A bioterrorism agent?

A. *Anaplasma phagocytophilum*

B. *Bacillus cereus*

C. *Brucella melitensis*

D. *Coxiella burnetii*

E. *Francisella tularensis*

5. Which of the following drugs is the most appropriate treatment for this patient?

A. Penicillin

B. Streptomycin

C. Vancomycin

D. Erythromycin

E. Ceftriaxone

Answers and Explanations

1. Correct: *Yersinia pestis* (E)

Described is a case of bubonic plague, caused by *Yersinia pestis*. The patient lives in a geographic area where plague is endemic (south or southwestern United States) and he has been exposed to the reservoir (mice and other small rodents) within the previous 2 to 7 days before symptoms first appeared. Symptoms include sudden onset of fever and the presence of painful and swollen inguinal lymph nodes, termed buboes. In some cases, cervical or axillary lymph nodes may be involved. Furthermore, the causative agent is a gram-negative rod seen in the figure. Of note, *Y. pestis* often stain as bipolar bacilli on Wayson's or Wright's stain but are sometimes visualized on Gram stain (as shown in the figure). If untreated, this patient would be at risk of developing possible life-threatening pneumonic plague if the bacteria disseminate to the lungs. All of the other possible answer choices are zoonotic infections.

A *Bacillus anthracis* would more likely present as a black eschar, and the Gram stain would show large gram-positive rods with a characteristic boxcar shape.

B *Borrelia burgdorferi* is the causative agent of Lyme disease and is transmitted by ticks. The Gram stain of *B. burgdorferi* would show weekly gram-negative spirochetes, Although it is characterized as neither gram-negative or gram-positive. The clinical presentation would include an erythema migrans rash.

C *Coxiella burnetii* is the causative agent of Q fever and is an obligate intracellular gram-negative coccobacilli, not extracellular bacilli as are shown in the figure.

D *Francisella tularensis* is the causative agent of tularemia, which is more often associated with exposure to infected rabbits and do not grow on routine laboratory media.

2. Correct: Mice (D)

This patient has bubonic plague, caused by the bacteria *Y. pestis*. The rodent flea is the vector for *Y. pestis* and small mammals are the reservoirs: mice, squirrels, prairie dogs, rats, chipmunks, rabbits, etc. Infection is normally from a bite from the vector flea or handling infected animals. In this case, the patient most likely contracted the infection from the dead mice that he and his friends encountered in the woods.

A The bubonic form of the plague is not transmitted person to person; however, the pneumonic form may be transmitted by respiratory droplets. Therefore, it is unlikely that this patient could have developed bubonic plague from a fellow camper.

B Horses are not known reservoirs for this infection.

C *Y. pestis* is a zoonotic infection. The vector is the rodent flea, not the mosquito.

E The pond is not a likely source of *Y. pestis*. These bacteria are unable to form spores and are therefore not likely to be able to survive in the environment. .

3. Correct: Lipopolysaccharide (LPS) (B)

This case describes bubonic plague, caused by *Y. pestis*. These bacteria normally enter the body via the subcutaneous route and a low infectious dose is required. They travel via the lymphatics to regional lymph nodes where most of the damage is caused by the host inflammatory response to the infection. As such, these bacteria do not produce many classical virulence factors. They are gram-negative, and as such, produce LPS on the surface, which is thought to contribute to the host immune response. In addition, *Y. pestis* is able to survive within macrophages, which may aid in the dissemination of the organism to the lymph nodes during infection.

A Exotoxin A is produced by *Pseudomonas aeruginosa*, and the mode of action is to kill host cells by ADP-ribosylation of elongation factor-2.

C Lipoteichoic acid is produced by most gram-positive bacteria, but *Y. pestis* is a gram-negative organism.

D Pili are produced by many bacteria and usually facilitate adhesion, or are involved in gene exchange via conjugation. While *Yersinia enterocolitica* produces a type IV pilus, there is no evidence for pili production by *Y. pestis*. *Y. pestis* adheres to host cells via nonpilus adhesin proteins.

E There is no evidence for a *Y. pestis* urease enzyme. Urease is produced by some gram-negative pathogens such as *Helicobacter pylori*.

4. Correct: *Francisella tularensis* (E)

This case describes a *Y. pestis* infection, bubonic plague. The airborne form of *Y. pestis* infection causes pneumonic plague, which is a highly transmissible infection with a high mortality rate. As a result, the CDC lists *Y. pestis* as a category A agent due to the high priority of this agent's lethality and transmissibility. The category A agents are plague, smallpox, tularemia, and the viral hemorrhagic fevers (i.e., Ebola, Marburg, etc.). Tularemia is caused by the bacteria *F. tularensis* (the correct answer to this question).

A, B, C, D Category B agents are moderately easy to disseminate and result in moderate morbidity rates and low mortality rates. Some category B agents include *Brucella melitensis, Coxiella burnetii,* and food or water safety threats. Both *Anaplasma phagocytophilum* and *Bacillus cereus* are not listed as CDC select agents.

5. Correct: Streptomycin (B)

The choices of treatment for plague are limited, but the antibiotic with the best supporting data is streptomycin. Other drug choices include gentamicin, levofloxacin, ciprofloxacin, doxycycline, and chloramphenicol which are not generally available in the United States.

A, C, D, E None of the other options listed are appropriate for treating *Y. pestis.*

Keywords: *Yersinia pestis*, bubonic plague, streptomycin, category A agent, lipopolysaccharide

Bibliography

Case 1

Aoyama T, Takeuchi Y, Goto A, Iwai H, Murase Y, Iwata T. Pertussis in adults. Am J Dis Child 1992;146(2):163–166

Murray P, Rosenthal K, Pfaller M. Medical Microbiology. Chapter 32: Bordetella. 7th ed. Saunders an imprint of Elsevier Inc; 2013

Wang K, Bettiol S, Thompson MJ, et al. Symptomatic treatment of the cough in whooping cough. Cochrane Database Syst Rev 2014;9(9):CD003257

Case 2

Fox JP, Hall CE, Cooney MK. The Seattle Virus Watch. VII. Observations of adenovirus infections. Am J Epidemiol 1977;105(4):362-386

Lynch JP 3rd, Kajon AE. Adenovirus: epidemiology, global spread of novel serotypes, and advances in treatment and prevention. Semin Respir Crit Care Med 2016;37(4):586–602

Pabbaraju K, Wong S, Fox JD. Detection of adenoviruses. Methods Mol Biol 2011;665:1–15

Sambursky R, Trattler W, Tauber S, et al. Sensitivity and specificity of the AdenoPlus test for diagnosing adenoviral conjunctivitis. JAMA Ophthalmol 2013;131(1):17–22

Case 3

Brocato RL, Hammerbeck CD, Bell TM, Wells JB, Queen LA, Hooper JW. A lethal disease model for hantavirus pulmonary syndrome in immunosuppressed Syrian hamsters infected with Sin Nombre virus. J Virol 2014;88(2):811–819

Hjelle B, Glass GE. Outbreak of hantavirus infection in the Four Corners region of the United States in the wake of the 1997–1998 El Nino-southern oscillation. J Infect Dis 2000;181(5):1569çç1573

Machado AM, de Figueiredo GG, Sabino dos Santos G Jr, Figueiredo LTM. Laboratory diagnosis of human hantavirus infection: novel insights and future potential. Future Virol 2009;4:383–389

MacNeil A, Ksiazek TG, Rollin PE. Hantavirus pulmonary syndrome, United States, 1993-2009. Emerg Infect Dis 2011;17(7):1195–1201

Vapalahti O, Mustonen J, Lundkvist A, Henttonen H, Plyusnin A, Vaheri A. Hantavirus infections in Europe. Lancet Infect Dis 2003;3(10):653–661

Wernly JA, Dietl CA, Tabe CE, et al. Extracorporeal membrane oxygenation support improves survival of patients with Hantavirus cardiopulmonary syndrome refractory to medical treatment. Eur J Cardiothorac Surg 2011;40(6):1334–1340

Yoshimatsu K, Arikawa J. Serological diagnosis with recombinant N antigen for hantavirus infection. Virus Res 2014;187:77–83

Case 4

Baron EJ, Miller JM, Weinstein MP, et al. A guide to utilization of the microbiology laboratory for diagnosis of infectious diseases: 2013 recommendations by the Infectious Diseases Society of America (IDSA) and the American Society for Microbiology (ASM)(a). Clin Infect Dis 2013;57(4):e22–e121

Barsumian EL, Schlievert PM, Watson DW. Nonspecific and specific immunological mitogenicity by group A streptococcal pyrogenic exotoxins. Infect Immun 1978;22(3):681–688

Choby BA. Diagnosis and treatment of streptococcal pharyngitis. Am Fam Physician 2009;79(5):383–390

Edmonson MB, Farwell KR. Relationship between the clinical likelihood of group a streptococcal pharyngitis and the sensitivity of a rapid antigen-detection test in a pediatric practice. Pediatrics 2005;115(2):280–285

Gerber MA, Baltimore RS, Eaton CB, et al. Prevention of rheumatic fever and diagnosis and treatment of acute Streptococcal pharyngitis: a scientific statement from the American Heart Association Rheumatic Fever, Endocarditis, and Kawasaki Disease Committee of the Council on Cardiovascular Disease in the Young, the Interdisciplinary Council on Functional Genomics and Translational Biology, and the Interdisciplinary Council on Quality of Care and Outcomes Research: endorsed by the American Academy of Pediatrics. Circulation 2009;119(11):1541–1551

Guilherme L, Cunha-Neto E, Coelho V, et al. Human heart-infiltrating T-cell clones from rheumatic heart disease patients recognize both streptococcal and cardiac proteins. Circulation 1995;92(3):415–420

Peterson PK, Schmeling D, Cleary PP, Wilkinson BJ, Kim Y, Quie PG. Inhibition of alternative complement pathway opsonization by group A streptococcal M protein. J Infect Dis 1979;139(5):575–585

Shaikh N, Swaminathan N, Hooper EG. Accuracy and precision of the signs and symptoms of streptococcal pharyngitis in children: a systematic review. J Pediatr 2012;160(3):487–493.e3

Shulman ST, Bisno AL, Clegg HW, et al; Infectious Diseases Society of America. Clinical practice guideline for the diagnosis and management of group A streptococcal pharyngitis: 2012 update by the Infectious Diseases Society of America. Clin Infect Dis 2012;55(10):e86–e102

Stevens DL. Streptococcus pyogenes Infections. In: Stein JH, ed. Internal Medicine. 4th ed. St. Louis, MO: Mosby; 1994:2078

Case 5

Murray P, Rosenthal K, Pfaller M. Medical Microbiology. Chapter 24: Haemophilus and related bacteria. 7th ed. Saunders an imprint of Elsevier Inc; 2013

Plaut AG. The IgA1 proteases of pathogenic bacteria. Annu Rev Microbiol 1983;37:603–622

Case 6

Blaschke AJ. Interpreting assays for the detection of Streptococcus pneumoniae. Clin Infect Dis 2011;52(Suppl 4):S331–S337

Centers for Disease Control and Prevention (CDC). Recommended child and adolescent immunization schedule for ages 18 years or younger, United States, 2019. Available at: https://www.cdc.gov/vaccines/schedules/hcp/imz/child-adolescent.html. Accessed December 11, 2019

Gutiérrez F, Masiá M, Rodríguez JC, et al. Evaluation of the immunochromatographic Binax NOW assay for detection of Streptococcus pneumoniae urinary antigen in a prospective study of community-acquired pneumonia in Spain. Clin Infect Dis 2003;36(3):286–292

Heffron R. Pneumonia, with Special Reference to Pneumococcus Lobar Pneumonia. New York, NY: Commonwealth Fund;1939

Kobayashi M. Intervals between PCV13 and PPSV23 vaccines: evidence supporting currently recommended intervals and proposed changes. Advisory Committee on Immunization Practices, June 25, 2015. Available at: http://www.cdc.gov/vaccines/acip/meetings/downloads/slides-2015-06/pneumo-02-kobayashi.pdf. Accessed August 03, 2015

Metlay JP, Schulz R, Li YH, et al. Influence of age on symptoms at presentation in patients with community-acquired pneumonia. Arch Intern Med 1997;157(13):1453-1459

Moore MR, Link-Gelles R, Schaffner W, et al. Effect of use of 13-valent pneumococcal conjugate vaccine in children on invasive pneumococcal disease in children and adults in the USA: analysis of multisite, population-based surveillance. Lancet Infect Dis 2015;15(3):301–309

Rosón B, Fernández-Sabé N, Carratalà J, et al. Contribution of a urinary antigen assay (Binax NOW) to the early diagnosis of pneumococcal pneumonia. Clin Infect Dis 2004;38(2):222–226

Tomasz A, Albino A, Zanati E. Multiple antibiotic resistance in a bacterium with suppressed autolytic system. Nature 1970;227(5254):138–140

Case 7

Burillo A, Pedro-Botet MLBE, Bouza E. Microbiology and epidemiology of Legionnaire's disease. Infect Dis Clin North Am 2017;31(1):7–27

Mandell LA, Wunderink RG, Anzueto A, et al; Infectious Diseases Society of America; American Thoracic Society. Infectious Diseases Society of America/American Thoracic Society consensus guidelines on the management of community-acquired pneumonia in adults. Clin Infect Dis 2007;44(Suppl 2):S27–S72

Misch EA. Legionella: virulence factors and host response. Curr Opin Infect Dis 2016;29(3):280–286

Yu VL, Plouffe JF, Pastoris MC, et al. Distribution of Legionella species and serogroups isolated by culture in patients with sporadic community-acquired legionellosis: an international collaborative survey. J Infect Dis 2002;186(1):127–128

Case 8

Li Z, Kosorok MR, Farrell PM, et al. Longitudinal development of mucoid Pseudomonas aeruginosa infection and lung disease progression in children with cystic fibrosis. JAMA 2005;293(5):581–588

Meluleni GJ, Grout M, Evans DJ, Pier GB. Mucoid Pseudomonas aeruginosa growing in a biofilm in vitro are killed by opsonic antibodies to the mucoid exopolysaccharide capsule but not by antibodies produced during chronic lung infection in cystic fibrosis patients. J Immunol 1995;155(4):2029–2038

Murray P, Rosenthal K, Pfaller M. Medical Microbiology. Chapter 27: Pseudomonas and related bacteria. 7th ed. Saunders an imprint of Elsevier Inc; 2013

O'Sullivan BP, Freedman SD. Cystic fibrosis. Lancet 2009;373(9678):1891–1904

Ryall B, Carrara M, Zlosnik JE, et al. PLoS One 2014;9(5):e96166

Case 9

Fisher MC, Koenig GL, White TJ, Taylor JW. Molecular and phenotypic description of Coccidioides posadasii sp. nov., previously recognized as the non-California population of Coccidioides immitis. Mycologia 2002;94(1):73–84

Galgiani JN, Ampel NM, Blair JE, et al. 2016 Infectious Diseases Society of America (IDSA) Clinical Practice Guideline for the Treatment of Coccidioidomycosis. Clin Infect Dis 2016;63(6):e112–e146

Stevens DA, Clemons KV, Levine HB, et al. Expert opinion: what to do when there is Coccidioides exposure in a laboratory. Clin Infect Dis 2009;49(6):919–923

Umeyama T, Sano A, Kamei K, Niimi M, Nishimura K, Uehara Y. Novel approach to designing primers for identification and distinction of the human pathogenic fungi Coccidioides immitis and Coccidioides posadasii by PCR amplification. J Clin Microbiol 2006;44(5):1859–1862

Wieden MA, Lundergan LL, Blum J, et al. Detection of coccidioidal antibodies by 33-kDa spherule antigen, Coccidioides EIA, and standard serologic tests in sera from patients evaluated for coccidioidomycosis. J Infect Dis 1996;173(5):1273–1277

Case 10

Fuller H, Del Mar C. Immunoglobulin treatment for respiratory syncytial virus infection. Cochrane Database Syst Rev 2006;(4):CD004883

George-Gay B, Parker K. Understanding the complete blood count with differential. J Perianesth Nurs 2003;18(2):96–114, quiz 115–117

Hacking D, Hull J. Respiratory syncytial virus-viral biology and the host response. J Infect 2002;45(1):18–24

Krzyzaniak MA, Zumstein MT, Gerez JA, Picotti P, Helenius A. Host cell entry of respiratory syncytial virus involves macropinocytosis followed by proteolytic activation of the F protein. PLoS Pathog 2013;9(4):e1003309

Mastrangelo P, Hegele RG. RSV fusion: time for a new model. Viruses 2013;5(3):873–885

Sáez-Llorens X, Moreno MT, Ramilo O, Sánchez PJ, Top FH Jr, Connor EM; MEDI-493 Study Group. Safety and pharmacokinetics of palivizumab therapy in children hospitalized with respiratory syncytial virus infection. Pediatr Infect Dis J 2004;23(8):707–712

Ventre K, Randolph A. Ribavirin for respiratory syncytial virus infection of the lower respiratory tract in infants and young children. Cochrane Database Syst Rev 2004;(4):CD000181

Case 11

Belshe RB, Nichol KL, Black SB, et al. Safety, efficacy, and effectiveness of live, attenuated, cold-adapted influenza vaccine in an indicated population aged 5-49 years. Clin Infect Dis 2004;39(7):920–927

Clark A, Potter CW, Jennings R, et al. A comparison of live and inactivated influenza A (H1N1) virus vaccines. 2. Long-term immunity. J Hyg (Lond) 1983;90(3):361-370

Sasaki S, Sullivan M, Narvaez CF, et al. Limited efficacy of inactivated influenza vaccine in elderly individuals is associated with decreased production of vaccine-specific antibodies. J Clin Invest 2011;121(8):3109–3119

Sridhar S, Brokstad KA, Cox RJ. Influenza vaccination strategies: comparing inactivated and live attenuated influenza vaccines. Vaccines (Basel) 2015;3(2):373–389

van der Sluijs KF, van der Poll T, Lutter R, Juffermans NP, Schultz MJ. Bench-to-bedside review: bacterial pneumonia with influenza - pathogenesis and clinical implications. Crit Care 2010;14(2):219

van Elden LJR, van Essen GA, Boucher CAB, et al. Clinical diagnosis of influenza virus infection: evaluation of diagnostic tools in general practice. Br J Gen Pract 2001;51(469):630–634

Case 12

Cahill TJ, Prendergast BD. Infective endocarditis. Lancet 2016;387(10021):882–893

Durack DT, Lukes AS, Bright DK; Duke Endocarditis Service. New criteria for diagnosis of infective endocarditis: utilization of specific echocardiographic findings. Am J Med 1994;96(3):200–209

Li JS, Sexton DJ, Mick N, et al. Proposed modifications to the Duke criteria for the diagnosis of infective endocarditis. Clin Infect Dis 2000;30(4):633–638

Murdoch DR, Corey GR, Hoen B, et al; International Collaboration on Endocarditis-Prospective Cohort Study (ICE-PCS) Investigators. Clinical presentation, etiology, and outcome of infective endocarditis in the 21st century: the International Collaboration on Endocarditis-Prospective Cohort Study. Arch Intern Med 2009;169(5):463–473

Case 13

Karmali MA, Petric M, Lim C, Fleming PC, Arbus GS, Lior H. The association between idiopathic hemolytic uremic syndrome and infection by verotoxin-producing Escherichia coli. J Infect Dis 1985;151(5):775–782

Slutsker L, Ries AA, Greene KD, Wells JG, Hutwagner L, Griffin PM. Escherichia coli O157:H7 diarrhea in the United States: clinical and epidemiologic features. Ann Intern Med 1997;126(7):505–513

Su C, Brandt LJ. Escherichia coli O157:H7 infection in humans. Ann Intern Med 1995;123(9):698–714

Tarr PI, Gordon CA, Chandler WL. Shiga-toxin-producing Escherichia coli and haemolytic uraemic syndrome. Lancet 2005;365(9464):1073–1086

Tarr PI, Neill MA, Clausen CR, Watkins SL, Christie DL, Hickman RO. Escherichia coli O157:H7 and the hemolytic uremic syndrome: importance of early cultures in establishing the etiology. J Infect Dis 1990;162(2):553–556

Case 14

Bremell T, Bjelle A, Svedhem A. Rheumatic symptoms following an outbreak of campylobacter enteritis: a five year follow up. Ann Rheum Dis 1991;50(12):934–938

Centers for Disease Control and Prevention (CDC). Campylobacter jejuni infection associated with unpasteurized milk and cheese-Kansas, 2007. MMWR Morb Mortal Wkly Rep 2009;57(51):1377–1379

Chomel BB. Emerging and re-emerging zoonoses of dogs and cats. Animals (Basel) 2014;4(3):434–445

Jagusztyn-Krynicka EK, Łaniewski P, Wyszyńska A. Update on Campylobacter jejuni vaccine development for preventing human campylobacteriosis. Expert Rev Vaccines 2009;8(5):625–645

Nachamkin I, Allos BM, Ho T. Campylobacter species and Guillain-Barré syndrome. Clin Microbiol Rev 1998;11(3): 555–567

Rees JR, Pannier MA, McNees A, Shallow S, Angulo FJ, Vugia DJ. Persistent diarrhea, arthritis, and other complications of enteric infections: a pilot survey based on California FoodNet surveillance, 1998-1999. Clin Infect Dis 2004;38(Suppl 3): S311–S317

Case 15

Beuret C. Simultaneous detection of enteric viruses by multiplex real-time RT-PCR. J Virol Methods 2004;115(1):1–8

Freeland AL, Vaughan GH Jr, Banerjee SN. Acute Gastroenteritis on Cruise Ships-United States, 2008-2014. MMWR Morb Mortal Wkly Rep 2016;65(1):1–5

Hall AJ, Lopman BA, Payne DC, et al. Norovirus disease in the United States. Emerg Infect Dis 2013;19(8):1198–1205

Hall AJ, Wikswo ME, Pringle K, Gould LH, Parashar UD; Division of Viral Diseases, National Center for Immunization and Respiratory Diseases, CDC. Vital signs: foodborne norovirus outbreaks-United States, 2009-2012. MMWR Morb Mortal Wkly Rep 2014;63(22):491–495

Lambden PR, Caul EO, Ashley CR, Clarke IN. Sequence and genome organization of a human small round-structured (Norwalk-like) virus. Science 1993;259(5094):516–519

Case 16

Bartlett JG. Narrative review: the new epidemic of Clostridium difficile-associated enteric disease. Ann Intern Med 2006;145(10): 758–764

Gerding DN, Johnson S, Peterson LR, Mulligan ME, Silva J Jr. Clostridium difficile-associated diarrhea and colitis. Infect Control Hosp Epidemiol 1995;16(8):459–477

Kim KH, Fekety R, Batts DH, et al. Isolation of Clostridium difficile from the environment and contacts of patients with antibiotic-associated colitis. J Infect Dis 1981;143(1):42–50

Leffler DA, Lamont JT. Clostridium difficile infection. N Engl J Med 2015;372(16):1539–1548

Price SB, Phelps CJ, Wilkins TD, Johnson JL. Cloning of the carbohydrate-binding portion of the toxin a gene of Clostridium difficile. Curr Microbiol 1987;16:55

Case 17

Agholi M, Hatam GR, Motazedian MH. HIV/AIDS-associated opportunistic protozoal diarrhea. AIDS Res Hum Retroviruses 2013;29(1):35–41

Esfandiari A, Swartz J, Teklehaimanot S. Clustering of giardiosis among AIDS patients in Los Angeles County. Cell Mol Biol 1997;43(7):1077–1083

Kumar T, Abd Majid MA, Onichandran S, et al. Presence of Cryptosporidium parvum and Giardia lamblia in water samples from Southeast Asia: towards an integrated water detection system. Infect Dis Poverty 2016;5:3

Levine GI. Sexually transmitted parasitic diseases. Prim Care 1991;18(1):101–128

Case 18

Chen SL, Morgan TR. The natural history of hepatitis C virus (HCV) infection. Int J Med Sci 2006;3(2):47–52

Chiu WC, Tsan YT, Tsai SL, Chang CJ, Wang JD, Chen PC; Health Data Analysis in Taiwan (hDATa) Research Group. Hepatitis C viral infection and the risk of dementia. Eur J Neurol 2014;21(8):1068–e59

de Oliveria Andrade LJ, D'Oliveira A, Melo RC, De Souza EC, Costa Silva CA, Paraná R. Association between hepatitis C and hepatocellular carcinoma. J Glob Infect Dis 2009;1(1):33–37

Spengler U, Nattermann J. Immunopathogenesis in hepatitis C virus cirrhosis. Clin Sci (Lond) 2007;112(3):141–155

Tohme RA, Holmberg SD. Transmission of hepatitis C virus infection through tattooing and piercing: a critical review. Clin Infect Dis 2012;54(8):1167–1178 Available at: http://hcvguidelines.org. Accessed August 6, 2019

Case 19

Cai YJ, Dong JJ, Wang XD, et al. A diagnostic algorithm for assessment of liver fibrosis by liver stiffness measurement in patients with chronic hepatitis B. J Viral Hepat 2017;24(11):1005–1015

Chang ML, Liaw YF. Hepatitis B flares in chronic hepatitis B: pathogenesis, natural course, and management. J Hepatol 2014;61(6):1407–1417

D'Souza R, Foster GR. Diagnosis and treatment of chronic hepatitis B. J R Soc Med 2004;97(7):318–321

Gonzalez SA, Perrillo RP, Hepatitis B. Hepatitis B virus reactivation in the setting of cancer chemotherapy and other immunosuppressive drug therapy. Clin Infect Dis 2016;62(Suppl 4):S306–S313

Kim HY, Kim W. Chemotherapy-related reactivation of hepatitis B infection: updates in 2013. World J Gastroenterol 2014;20(40):14581–14588

Liang TJ, Hepatitis B. Hepatitis B: the virus and disease. Hepatology 2009;49(5, Suppl):S13–S21

U.S. Department of Health and Human Services. Office of Minority Health, Minority Population Profiles. Available from: https://minorityhealth.hhs.gov/omh/browse.aspx?lvl=4&lvlid=50. Accessed August 6, 2019

Yeo W, Johnson PJ. Diagnosis, prevention and management of hepatitis B virus reactivation during anticancer therapy. Hepatology 2006;43(2):209–220

Case 20

Calvet X, Sánchez-Delgado J, Montserrat A, et al. Accuracy of diagnostic tests for Helicobacter pylori: a reappraisal. Clin Infect Dis 2009;48(10):1385–1391

Goodwin CS, Worsley BW. Microbiology of Helicobacter pylori. Gastroenterol Clin North Am 1993;22(1):5–19

Kao CY, Sheu BS, Wu JJ. Helicobacter pylori infection: an overview of bacterial virulence factors and pathogenesis. Biomed J 2016;39(1):14–23

NIH Consensus Conference. Helicobacter pylori in peptic ulcer disease. NIH Consensus Development Panel on Helicobacter pylori in Peptic Ulcer Disease. JAMA 1994;272(1):65–69

Case 21

Griffith DP. Struvite stones. Kidney Int 1978;13(5):372–382

Madigan Michael T, Martinko John M, Bender Kelly S, Buckley Daniel H, Stahl David A, Brock Thomas. Brock Biology of Microorganisms. 14th ed. Harlow, UK: Pearson; 2015

Mobley HL, Island MD, Massad G. Virulence determinants of uropathogenic Escherichia coli and Proteus mirabilis. Kidney Int Suppl 1994;47:S129–S136

Murray Patrick R, Rosenthal Ken S, Pfaller Michael A. Enterobacteriaceae. Medical Microbiology. 2016:251–264.e1

Preminger Glenn M, Curhan Gary C. Pathogenesis and clinical manifestations of struvite stones. UpToDate. 2016

Case 22

Binnicker MJ, Jespersen DJ, Rollins LO. Treponema-specific tests for serodiagnosis of syphilis: comparative evaluation of seven assays. J Clin Microbiol 2011;49(4):1313–1317

Cantor AG, Pappas M, Daeges M, Nelson HD. Screening for syphilis: updated evidence report and systematic review for the us preventive services task force. JAMA 2016;315(21):2328–2337

Causer LM, Kaldor JM, Fairley CK, et al. A laboratory-based evaluation of four rapid point-of-care tests for syphilis. PLoS One 2014;9(3):e91504

Hallmark CJ, Hill MJ, Luswata C, et al. Déjà vu? A comparison of syphilis outbreaks in Houston, Texas. Sex Transm Dis 2016;43(9):549–555

Hook EW. Syphilis. Lancet 2017;389 (10078):1550–1557

Case 23

Centers for Disease Control and Prevention. Recommendations for the laboratory-based detection of Chlamydia trachomatis and Neisseria gonorrhoeae-2014. MMWR Recomm Rep 2014;63:1

Handsfield HH, Sparling PF. Neisseria gonorrhoeae. In: Mandell GL, Bennett JE, Dolin R, eds. Principles and Practice of Infectious Diseases. 4th ed. New York, NY: Churchill Livingstone; 1995:1909

Komaroff AL, Aronson MD, Pass TM, Ervin CT. Prevalence of pharyngeal gonorrhea in general medical patients with sore throats. Sex Transm Dis 1980;7(3):116–119

O'Brien JP, Goldenberg DL, Rice PA. Disseminated gonococcal infection: a pro-spective analysis of 49 patients and a review of pathophysiology and immune mechanisms. Medicine (Baltimore) 1983; 62(6):395–406

Rothbard JB, Fernandez R, Wang L, Teng NN, Schoolnik GK. Antibodies to peptides corresponding to a conserved sequence of gonococcal pilins block bacterial adhesion. Proc Natl Acad Sci U S A 1985;82(3):915–919

Wiesner PJ, Tronca E, Bonin P, Pedersen AH, Holmes KK. Clinical spectrum of pharyngeal gonococcal infection. N Engl J Med 1973;288(4):181–185

Case 24

Davis JP, Osterholm MT, Helms CM, et al. Tri-state toxic-shock syndrome study. II. Clinical and laboratory findings. J Infect Dis 1982;145(4):441–448

Lehn N, Schaller E, Wagner H, Krönke M. Frequency of toxic shock syndrome toxin- and enterotoxin-producing clinical isolates of Staphylococcus aureus. Eur J Clin Microbiol Infect Dis 1995;14(1):43–46

Parsonnet J. Mediators in the pathogenesis of toxic shock syndrome: overview. Rev Infect Dis 1989;11(Suppl 1):S263–S269

Reingold AL, Dan BB, Shands KN, Broome CV. Toxic-shock syndrome not associated with menstruation. A review of 54 cases. Lancet 1982;1(8262):1–4

Schlievert PM. Role of superantigens in human disease. J Infect Dis 1993;167(5):997–1002

Toxic Shock Syndrome (other than streptococcal) (TSS) 2011 Case Definition. http://wwwn.cdc.gov/nndss/conditions/toxic-shock-syndrome-other-than-streptococcal/case-definition/2011/. Accessed August 25, 2015

Case 25

Ernst AA, Marvez-Valls E, Martin DH. Incision and drainage versus aspiration of fluctuant buboes in the emergency department during an epidemic of chancroid. Sex Transm Dis 1995;22(4):217–220

González-Beiras C, Marks M, Chen CY, Roberts S, Mitjà O. Epidemiology of Haemophilus ducreyi infections. Emerg Infect Dis 2016;22(1):1–8 https://www.cdc.gov/std/tg2015/chancroid.htm. Accessed August 27, 2019

Lewis DA, Mitjà O. Haemophilus ducreyi: from sexually transmitted infection to skin ulcer pathogen. Curr Opin Infect Dis 2016;29(1):52–57

Weiss HA, Thomas SL, Munabi SK, Hayes RJ. Male circumcision and risk of syphilis, chancroid, and genital herpes: a systematic review and meta-analysis. Sex Transm Infect 2006;82(2):101–109, discussion 110

Case 26

Anger HA, Proops D, Harris TG, et al. Active Case finding and prevention of tuberculosis among a cohort of contacts exposed to infectious tuberculosis cases in New York City. Clin Infect Dis 2012;54(9):1287–1295

Centers for Disease Control and Prevention (CDC). Quick reference guide - Laboratory testing for the diagnosis of HIV infection : updated recommendations United States, 2014. Available at: https://stacks.cdc.gov/view/cdc/23446. Accessed December 11, 2019

Jensen PA, Lambert LA, Iademarco MF, Ridzon R; CDC. Guidelines for preventing the transmission of Mycobacterium tuberculosis in health-care settings, 2005. MMWR Recomm Rep 2005;54(RR-17):1–141

Kent PT, Kubica GP. Public Health Mycobacteriology: A Guide for the Level III Laboratory. Atlanta, GA: Centers for Disease Control, US PHS; 1985

Koneman EW, Allen SD, Janda WM, et al. Color Atlas and Textbook of Diagnostic Microbiology. Philadelphia, PA: Lippincott; 1997

McKinney JD, Höner zu Bentrup K, Muñoz-Elías EJ, et al. Persistence of Mycobacterium tuberculosis in macrophages and mice requires the glyoxylate shunt enzyme isocitrate lyase. Nature 2000;406(6797):735–738

Rastogi N, David HL. Mechanisms of pathogenicity in mycobacteria. Biochimie 1988;70(8):1101–1120

Reimer LG, Carroll KC. Role of the microbiology laboratory in the diagnosis of lower respiratory tract infections. Clin Infect Dis 1998;26(3):742–748

Case 27

Bhattar S, Bhalla P, Rawat D, Tripathi R, Kaur R, Sardana K. Correlation of CD4 T cell count and plasma viral load with reproductive tract infections/sexually transmitted infections in HIV infected females. J Clin Diagn Res 2014;8(10):DC12-DC14

Lloyd SB, Kent SJ, Winnall WR. The high cost of fidelity. AIDS Res Hum Retroviruses 2014;30(1):8–16

Lortholary O, Petrikkos G, Akova M, et al; ESCMID Fungal Infection Study Group. ESCMID* guideline for the diagnosis and management of Candida diseases 2012: patients with HIV infection or AIDS. Clin Microbiol Infect 2012;18(Suppl 7):68–77

Merenstein D, Hu H, Wang C, et al. Colonization by Candida species of the oral and vaginal mucosa in HIV-infected and noninfected women. AIDS Res Hum Retroviruses 2013;29(1):30–34

Case 28

Butler TKH, Spencer NA, Chan CCK, Singh Gilhotra J, McClellan K. Infective keratitis in older patients: a 4 year review, 1998-2002. Br J Ophthalmol 2005;89(5):591–596

Freeman ML, Sheridan BS, Bonneau RH, Hendricks RL. Psychological stress compromises CD8+ T cell control of latent herpes simplex virus type 1 infections. J Immunol 2007;179(1):322–328

Kaye S, Choudhary A. Herpes simplex keratitis. Prog Retin Eye Res 2006;25(4):355–380

Case 29

Centers for Disease Control and Prevention (CDC). STD Treatment Guidelines. Available at: https://www.cdc.gov/std/tg2015/warts.htm. Accessed August 28, 2019.

Egawa N, Doorbar J. The low-risk papillomaviruses. Virus Res 2017;231:119–127

Karnes JB, Usatine RP. Management of external genital warts. Am Fam Physician 2014;90(5):312–318

Ramakrishnan S, Partricia S, Mathan G. Overview of high-risk HPV's 16 and 18 infected cervical cancer: pathogenesis to prevention. Biomed Pharmacother 2015;70(C):103–110

Yanofsky VR, Patel RV, Goldenberg G. Genital warts: a comprehensive review. J Clin Aesthet Dermatol 2012;5(6):25–36 Available at: http://www.pubmedcentral.nih.gov/articlerender.fcgi?artid=3390234&tool=pmcentrez&rendertype=abstract. Accessed August 28, 2019

Case 30

David R, Barron BJ, Madewell JE. Osteomyelitis, acute and chronic. Radiol Clin North Am 1987;25(6):1171–1201

Lew DP, Waldvogel FA. Osteomyelitis. N Engl J Med 1997;336(14):999–1007

Miller LG, Diep BA. Clinical practice: colonization, fomites, and virulence: rethinking the pathogenesis of community-associated methicillin-resistant Staphylococcus aureus infection. Clin Infect Dis 2008;46(5):752–760

Naimi TS, LeDell KH, Como-Sabetti K, et al. Comparison of community- and health care-associated methicillin-resistant Staphylococcus aureus infection. JAMA 2003;290(22):2976–2984

Panton PN, Valentine FCO. Staphylococcal toxin. Lancet 1932;1:506

Patzakis MJ, Rao S, Wilkins J, Moore TM, Harvey PJ. Analysis of 61 cases of vertebral osteomyelitis. Clin Orthop Relat Res 1991; (264):178–183

Case 31

Anaya DA, Dellinger EP. Necrotizing soft-tissue infection: diagnosis and management. Clin Infect Dis 2007;44(5):705–710

Brook I, Frazier EH. Clinical and microbiological features of necrotizing fasciitis. J Clin Microbiol 1995;33(9):2382–2387

Chelsom J, Halstensen A, Haga T, Høiby EA. Necrotising fasciitis due to group A streptococci in western Norway: incidence and clinical features. Lancet 1994; 344(8930):1111–1115

Darenberg J, Luca-Harari B, Jasir A, et al. Molecular and clinical characteristics of invasive group A streptococcal infection in Sweden. Clin Infect Dis 2007;45(4):450–458

Facklam RR, Padula JF, Thacker LG, Wortham EC, Sconyers BJ. Presumptive identification of group A, B, and D streptococci. Appl Microbiol 1974;27(1):107–113

Schwartz MN, Pasternack MS. Cellulitis and subcutaneous tissue infections. In: Mandell GL, Bennett JE, Dolin R, eds. Principles and Practice of Infectious Diseases. 6th ed. Philadelphia, PA: Churchill Livingstone; 2005:1172

Shulman ST, Stollerman G, Beall B, Dale JB, Tanz RR. Temporal changes in streptococcal M protein types and the near-disappearance of acute rheumatic fever in the United States. Clin Infect Dis 2006;42(4):441–447

Singh G, Sinha SK, Adhikary S, Babu KS, Ray P, Khanna SK. Necrotising infections of soft tissues-a clinical profile. Eur J Surg 2002;168(6):366–371

Wong CH, Chang HC, Pasupathy S, Khin LW, Tan JL, Low CO. Necrotizing fasciitis: clinical presentation, microbiology, and determinants of mortality. J Bone Joint Surg Am 2003;85(8):1454–1460

Case 32

Gorbach SL, Thadepalli H. Isolation of Clostridium in human infections: evaluation of 114 cases. J Infect Dis 1975;131(Suppl):S81–S85

Lorber B. Gas gangrene and other Clostridium-associated diseases. In: Mandell GL, Bennett JE, Dolin R, eds. Principles and Practice of Infectious Diseases. 6th ed. Philadelphia, PA: Churchill Livingstone; 2005:2828

McNee JW, Dunn JS. The method of spread of gas gangrene into living muscle. Br Med J 1917;1:726.4–729

Stevens DL, Bisno AL, Chambers HF, et al; Infectious Diseases Society of America. Practice guidelines for the diagnosis and management of skin and soft tissue infections: 2014 update by the Infectious Diseases Society of America. Clin Infect Dis 2014;59(2):e10–e52

Stevens DL, Titball RW, Jepson M, Bayer CR, Hayes-Schroer SM, Bryant AE. Immunization with the C-Domain of alpha-Toxin prevents lethal infection, localizes tissue injury, and promotes host response to challenge with Clostridium perfringens. J Infect Dis 2004;190(4):767–773

Stevens DL, Tweten RK, Awad MM, Rood JI, Bryant AE. Clostridial gas gangrene: evidence that alpha and theta toxins differentially modulate the immune response and induce acute tissue necrosis. J Infect Dis 1997;176(1):189–195

Case 33

American College of Physicians. Guidelines for laboratory evaluation in the diagnosis of Lyme disease. Ann Intern Med 1997;127(12):1106–1108

Coulter P, Lema C, Flayhart D, et al. Two-year evaluation of Borrelia burgdorferi culture and supplemental tests for definitive diagnosis of Lyme disease. J Clin Microbiol 2005;43(10):5080–5084

Hyde JA, Trzeciakowski JP, Skare JT. Borrelia burgdorferi alters its gene expression and antigenic profile in response to CO2 levels. J Bacteriol 2007;189(2):437–445

Steere AC, Malawista SE, Snydman DR, et al. Lyme arthritis: an epidemic of oligoarticular arthritis in children and adults in three connecticut communities. Arthritis Rheum 1977;20(1):7–17

Steere AC, Sikand VK. The presenting manifestations of Lyme disease and the outcomes of treatment. N Engl J Med 2003;348(24):2472–2474

Takayama K, Rothenberg RJ, Barbour AG. Absence of lipopolysaccharide in the Lyme disease spirochete, Borrelia burgdorferi. Infect Immun 1987;55(9):2311–2313

Tugwell P, Dennis DT, Weinstein A, et al. Laboratory evaluation in the diagnosis of Lyme disease. Ann Intern Med 1997; 127(12):1109–1123

Wormser GP, Dattwyler RJ, Shapiro ED, et al. The clinical assessment, treatment, and prevention of lyme disease, human granulocytic anaplasmosis, and babesiosis: clinical practice guidelines by the Infectious Diseases Society of America. Clin Infect Dis 2006;43(9):1089–1134

Zückert WR. Laboratory maintenance of Borrelia burgdorferi. Curr Protoc Microbiol 2007

Case 34

Burgdorfer W, Anacker RL, Bird RG, Bertram DS. Intranuclear growth of Rickettsia rickettsii. J Bacteriol 1968;96(4):1415–1418

Cell J, Tsolis RM. Bacteria, the endoplasmic reticulum and the unfolded protein response: friends or foes? Nat Rev Microbiol 2015;13(2):71–82

Chapman AS, Bakken JS, Folk SM, et al; Tickborne Rickettsial Diseases Working Group; CDC. Diagnosis and management of tickborne rickettsial diseases: Rocky Mountain spotted fever, ehrlichioses, and anaplasmosis-United States: a practical guide for physicians and other health-care and public health professionals. MMWR Recomm Rep 2006;55(RR-4):1–27

David H. Walker. Rickettsia rickettsii and other spotted fever group rickettsiae. In: Mandell G, Bennett J, Dolin R, eds. Principles and Practice of Infectious Diseases. 8th ed. Saunders an imprint of Elsevier; 2015: 2198-2205

Drexler NA, Dahlgren FS, Heitman KN, Massung RF, Paddock CD, Behravesh CB. National surveillance of spotted fever group rickettsioses in the United States, 2008-2012. Am J Trop Med Hyg 2016;94(1):26–34

McQuiston J. CDC Yellow Book. Chapter 3: Infectious disease related to travel. Rickettsial (Spotted and Typhus Fevers) and Related Infections (Anaplasmosis and Ehrlichiosis). Available at: https://

wwwnc.cdc.gov/travel/yellowbook/2016/ infectious-diseases-related-to-travel/ rickettsial-spotted-typhus-fevers-related-infections-anaplasmosis-ehrlichiosis. Accessed 29th August, 2019

Thorner AR, Walker DH, Petri WA Jr. Rocky mountain spotted fever. Clin Infect Dis 1998;27(6):1353-1359, quiz 1360

Case 35

Beaman BL, Black CM, Doughty F, Beaman L. Role of superoxide dismutase and catalase as determinants of pathogenicity of Nocardia asteroides: importance in resistance to microbicidal activities of human polymorphonuclear neutrophils. Infect Immun 1985;47(1):135–141

Conville PS, Witebsky FG. Nocardia, Rhodococcus, Gordonia, Actinomadura, Streptomyces, and other aerobic Actinomycetes. In: Murray PR, Baron EJ, Jorgensen JH, et al., eds. Manual of Clinical Microbiology. 9th ed. Washington, DC: ASM Press; 2007:515

Lerner PI. Nocardiosis. Clin Infect Dis 1996;22(6):891-903, quiz 904–905

Martínez Tomás R, Menéndez Villanueva R, Reyes Calzada S, et al. Pulmonary nocardiosis: risk factors and outcomes. Respirology 2007;12(3):394–400

McNeil MM, Brown JM. The medically important aerobic actinomycetes: epidemiology and microbiology. Clin Microbiol Rev 1994;7(3):357–417

Muricy EC, Lemes RA, Bombarda S, Ferrazoli L, Chimara E. Differentiation between Nocardia spp. and Mycobacterium spp.: critical aspects for bacteriological diagnosis. Rev Inst Med Trop São Paulo 2014;56(5): 397–401

Sorrel TC, Mitchell DH, Iredell JR, Chen SC-A. Nocardia species. In: Mandell GL, Bennett JE, Dolin R, eds. Principles and Practice of Infectious Diseases. 7th ed. Philadelphia, PA: Churchill Livingstone Elsevier; 2010:3199

Wilson JW. Nocardiosis: updates and clinical overview. Mayo Clin Proc 2012; 87(4):403–407

Case 36

Farmakiotis D, Kontoyiannis DP. Mucormycoses. Infect Dis Clin North Am 2016;30(1):143–163

Greenberg RN, Scott LJ, Vaughn HH, Ribes JA. Zygomycosis (mucormycosis): emerging clinical importance and new treatments. Curr Opin Infect Dis 2004;17(6):517–525

Ibrahim AS, Spellberg B, Walsh TJ, Kontoyiannis DP. Pathogenesis of mucormycosis. Clin Infect Dis 2012;54(Suppl 1): S16–S22

Kauffman CA, Malani AN. Zygomycosis: an emerging fungal infection with new options for management. Curr Infect Dis Rep 2007;9(6):435–440

Kontoyiannis DP. Decrease in the number of reported cases of zygomycosis among patients with diabetes mellitus: a hypothesis. Clin Infect Dis 2007;44(8):1089–1090

Maertens J, Demuynck H, Verbeken EK, et al. Mucormycosis in allogeneic bone marrow transplant recipients: report of five cases and review of the role of iron overload in the pathogenesis. Bone Marrow Transplant 1999;24(3):307–312

Nucci M, Marr KA. Emerging fungal diseases. Clin Infect Dis 2005;41(4):521–526

Petrikkos G, Skiada A, Lortholary O, Roilides E, Walsh TJ, Kontoyiannis DP. Epidemiology and clinical manifestations of mucormycosis. Clin Infect Dis 2012;54(Suppl 1):S23–S34

Rajagopalan S. Serious infections in elderly patients with diabetes mellitus. Clin Infect Dis 2005;40(7):990–996

Spellberg B, Ibrahim AS, Chin-Hong PV, et al. The Deferasirox-AmBisome Therapy for Mucormycosis (DEFEAT Mucor) study: a randomized, double-blinded, placebo-controlled trial. J Antimicrob Chemother 2012;67(3):715–722

Case 37

Barros MB, de Almeida Paes R, Schubach AO. Sporothrix schenckii and Sporotrichosis. Clin Microbiol Rev 2011;24(4):633–654

Dixon DM, Salkin IF, Duncan RA, et al. Isolation and characterization of Sporothrix schenckii from clinical and environmental sources associated with the largest U.S. epidemic of sporotrichosis. J Clin Microbiol 1991;29(6):1106–1113

Kauffman CA. Sporotrichosis. Clin Infect Dis 1999;29(2):231-236, quiz 237

Kwon-Chung KJ, Bennett JE. Sporotrichosis. In: Medical Mycology. Philadelphia, PA: Lea & Febiger; 1992:707

Reiss E. Cell wall composition. In: Howard DH, ed. Fungi Pathogenic for Humans and Animals, Part B: Pathogenicity and Detection. New York, NY: Marcel Dekker; 1985:57

Case 38

Johnson TL, Graham CB, Boegler KA, et al. Prevalence and diversity of tick-borne pathogens in nymphal Ixodes scapularis (Acari: Ixodidae) in Eastern National Parks. J Med Entomol 2017;54(3):742–751

Kowalski TJ, Jobe DA, Dolan EC, Kessler A, Lovrich SD, Callister SM. The emergence of clinically relevant babesiosis in Southwestern Wisconsin. WMJ 2015;114(4): 152–157

Vannier EG, Diuk-Wasser MA, Ben Mamoun C, Krause PJ. Babesiosis. Infect Dis Clin North Am 2015;29(2):357–370

Wormser GP, Dattwyler RJ, Shapiro ED, et al. The clinical assessment, treatment, and prevention of lyme disease, human granulocytic anaplasmosis, and babesiosis: clinical practice guidelines by the Infectious Diseases Society of America. Clin Infect Dis 2006;43(9):1089–1134

Case 39

Bayer-Garner IB. Monkeypox virus: histologic, immunohistochemical and electron-microscopic findings. J Cutan Pathol 2005;32(1):28–34

Nalca A, Rimoin AW, Bavari S, Whitehouse CA. Reemergence of monkeypox: prevalence, diagnostics, and countermeasures. Clin Infect Dis 2005;41(12):1765–1771

Reynolds MG, Davidson WB, Curns AT, et al. Spectrum of infection and risk factors for human monkeypox, United States, 2003. Emerg Infect Dis 2007;13(9):1332–1339

Weinstein RA, Nalca A, Rimoin AW, Bavari S, Whitehouse CA. Reemergence of monkeypox: prevalence, diagnostics, and countermeasures. Clin Infect Dis 2005;41(12):1765–1771

Case 40

Bester JC. Measles and measles vaccination: a review. JAMA Pediatr 2016;170(12): 1209–1215

Enanoria WT, Liu F, Zipprich J, et al. The effect of contact investigations and public health interventions in the control and prevention of measles transmission: a simulation study. PLoS One 2016;11(12):e0167160

Gahr P, DeVries AS, Wallace G, et al. An outbreak of measles in an undervaccinated community. Pediatrics 2014;134(1):e220–e228

Case 41

Bausch DG, Towner JS, Dowell SF, et al. Assessment of the risk of Ebola virus transmission from bodily fluids and fomites. J Infect Dis 2007;196(Suppl 2):S142–S147

Broadhurst MJ, Brooks TJG, Pollock NR. Diagnosis of Ebola virus disease: past, present, and future. Clin Microbiol Rev 2016;29(4):773–793

Feldmann H, Geisbert TW. Ebola haemorrhagic fever. Lancet 2011;377(9768):849–862

World Health Organization. Laboratory diagnosis of Ebola virus disease. Interim Guidel. September 19, 2014 Available at: https://www.iamat.org/country/sierra-leone/risk/malaria. Accessed September 9, 2019

Case 42

Centers for Disease Control and Prevention (CDC). Human rabies from exposure to a vampire bat in Mexico-Louisiana, 2010. MMWR Morb Mortal Wkly Rep 2011;60(31):1050–1052

Dietzschold B, Li J, Faber M, Schnell M. Concepts in the pathogenesis of rabies. Future Virol 2008;3(5):481–490

Dyer JL, Yager P, Orciari L, et al. Rabies surveillance in the United States during 2013. J Am Vet Med Assoc 2014;245(10):1111–1123

Ménager P, Roux P, Mégret F, et al. Toll-like receptor 3 (TLR3) plays a major role in the formation of rabies virus Negri Bodies. PLoS Pathog 2009;5(2):e1000315 1000315

Warrell MJ, Warrell DA. Rabies and other lyssavirus diseases. Lancet 2004; 363(9413):959–969

Zhang G, Fu ZF. Complete genome sequence of a street rabies virus from Mexico. J Virol 2012;86(19):10892–10893

Case 43

Borrow R, Alarcón P, Carlos J, et al. The Global Meningococcal Initiative: global epidemiology, the impact of vaccines on meningococcal disease and the importance of herd protection. Expert Rev Vaccines 2017;16(4):313–328

Centers for Disease Control and Prevention (CDC). Vaccines and Preventable Diseases: Meningococcal Vaccinaton. Available at: https://www.cdc.gov/vaccines/vpd/mening/index.html. Accessed September 2, 2019

Davis CE, Arnold K. Role of meningococcal endotoxin in meningococcal purpura. J Exp Med 1974;140(1):159-171

Hill DJ, Griffiths NJ, Borodina E, Virji M. Cellular and molecular biology of Neisseria meningitidis colonization and invasive disease. Clin Sci (Lond) 2010;118(9):547–564

Kim JH. A Challenge in vaccine development-Neisseria meningitidis serogroup B. N Engl J Med 2016;375(3):275–278

Klughammer J, Dittrich M, Blom J, et al. Comparative genome sequencing reveals within-host genetic changes in Neisseria meningitidis during invasive disease. PLoS One 2017;12(1):e0169892

Siddiqui R, Khan NA. Primary amoebic meningoencephalitis caused by Naegleria fowleri: an old enemy presenting new challenges. PLoS Negl Trop Dis 2014;8(8):e3017

Case 44

Bonazzi M, Lecuit M, Cossart P. Listeria monocytogenes internalin and E-cadherin: from bench to bedside. Cold Spring Harb Perspect Biol 2009;1(4):a003087

Cartwright EJ, Jackson KA, Johnson SD, Graves LM, Silk BJ, Mahon BE. Listeriosis outbreaks and associated food vehicles, United States, 1998-2008. Emerg Infect Dis 2013;19(1):1–9, quiz 184

Kearns DB. A field guide to bacterial swarming motility. Nat Rev Microbiol 2010;8(9):634–644

Lemon KP, Higgins DE, Kolter R. Flagellar motility is critical for Listeria monocytogenes biofilm formation. J Bacteriol 2007;189(12):4418–4424

Pagliano P, Ascione T, Boccia G, De Caro F, Esposito S. Listeria monocytogenes meningitis in the elderly: epidemiological, clinical and therapeutic findings. Infez Med 2016;24(2):105–111

Case 45

City NY, York N, Nile-like W, et al; Centers for Disease Control and Prevention (CDC). Outbreak of West Nile-like viral encephalitis-New York, 1999. MMWR Morb Mortal Wkly Rep 1999;48(38):845–849

Madden K. West Nile virus infection and its neurological manifestations. Clin Med Res 2003;1(2):145–150

Montgomery RR. Age-related alterations in immune responses to West Nile virus infection. Clin Exp Immunol 2017;187(1):26–34

Tunkel AR, Glaser CA, Bloch KC, et al. The management of encephalitis: clinical practice guidelines by the Infectious Diseases Society of America. Clin Infect Dis 2008;47(3):303–327

Tyler KL, Pape J, Goody RJ, Corkill M, Kleinschmidt-DeMasters BK. CSF findings in

250 patients with serologically confirmed West Nile virus meningitis and encephalitis. Neurology 2006;66(3):361–365

Case 46

Almeida F, Wolf JM, Casadevall A. Virulence-associated enzymes of Cryptococcus neoformans. Eukaryot Cell 2015;14(12):1173–1185

Buchanan KL, Murphy JW. What makes Cryptococcus neoformans a pathogen? Emerg Infect Dis 1998;4(1):71–83

Day JN, Chau TTH, Wolbers M, et al. Combination antifungal therapy for cryptococcal meningitis. N Engl J Med 2013;368(14):1291–1302

Pappas PG, Perfect JR, Cloud GA, et al. Cryptococcosis in human immunodeficiency virus-negative patients in the era of effective azole therapy. Clin Infect Dis 2001;33(5):690–699

Perfect JR, Dismukes WE, Dromer F, et al. Clinical practice guidelines for the management of cryptococcal disease: 2010 update by the Infectious Diseases Society of America. Clin Infect Dis 2010;50(3):291

Zaragoza O, Rodrigues ML, De Jesus M, Frases S, Dadachova E, Casadevall A. The capsule of the fungal pathogen Cryptococcus neoformans. Adv Appl Microbiol 2009;68:133–216

Case 47

Capewell LG, Harris AM, Yoder JS, et al. Diagnosis, clinical course, and treatment of primary amoebic meningoencephalitis in the United States, 1937–2013. J Pediatric Infect Dis Soc 2015;4(4):e68–e75

Siddiqui R, Ali IKM, Cope JR, Khan NA. Biology and pathogenesis of Naegleria fowleri. Acta Trop 2016;164:375-394

Siddiqui R, Khan NA. Primary amoebic meningoencephalitis caused by Naegleria fowleri: an old enemy presenting new challenges. PLoS Negl Trop Dis 2014;8(8):e3017

Yoder JS, Eddy BA, Visvesvara GS, Capewell L, Beach MJ. The epidemiology of primary amoebic meningoencephalitis in the USA, 1962-2008. Epidemiol Infect 2010;138(7):968–975

Case 48

Centers for Disease Control and Prevention (CDC). Rapid diagnostic tests for malaria-Haiti, 2010. MMWR Morb Mortal Wkly 2010;59(42):1372–1373

Centers for Disease Control and Prevention (CDC). Transmission of malaria in resort area-Dominican Republic, 2004. MMWR Morb Mortal Wkly 2005;53(51 & 52):1195–1198

Garcia JE, Puentes A, Patarroyo ME. Developmental biology of sporozoite-host interactions in Plasmodium falciparum malaria: implications for vaccine design. Clin Microbiol Rev 2006;19(4):686–707

Meibalan E, Marti M. Biology of malaria transmission. Cold Spring Harb Perspect Med 2017;7:a025452

Case 49

Bonalumi S, Trapanese A, Santamaria A, D'Emidio L, Mobili L. Cytomegalovirus infection in pregnancy: review of the literature. J Prenat Med 2011;5(1):1–8

Boppana SB, Ross SA, Novak Z, et al; National Institute on Deafness and Other Communication Disorders CMV and Hearing Multicenter Screening (CHIMES) Study. Dried blood spot real-time polymerase chain reaction assays to screen newborns for congenital cytomegalovirus infection. JAMA 2010;303(14):1375–1382

Kimberlin DW, Jester PM, Sánchez PJ, et al; National Institute of Allergy and Infectious Diseases Collaborative Antiviral Study Group. Valganciclovir for symptomatic congenital cytomegalovirus disease. N Engl J Med 2015;372(10):933–943

Kimberlin DW, Lin CY, Sánchez PJ, et al; National Institute of Allergy and Infectious Diseases Collaborative Antiviral Study Group. Effect of ganciclovir therapy on hearing in symptomatic congenital cytomegalovirus disease involving the central nervous system: a randomized, controlled trial. J Pediatr 2003;143(1):16–25

Oliver SE, Cloud GA, Sánchez PJ, et al; National Institute of Allergy, Infectious Diseases Collaborative Antiviral Study Group. Neurodevelopmental outcomes following ganciclovir therapy in symptomatic congenital cytomegalovirus infections involving the central nervous system. J Clin Virol 2009;46(Suppl 4):S22–S26

van Zuylen WJ, Hamilton ST, Naing Z, Hall B, Shand A, Rawlinson WD. Congenital cytomegalovirus infection: clinical presentation, epidemiology, diagnosis and prevention. Obstet Med 2014;7(4):140–146

Case 50

Centers for Disease Control and Prevention (CDC). Human plague-United States, 1993–1994. MMWR Morb Mortal Wkly Rep 1994;43(13):242–246

Collyn F, Léty MA, Nair S, et al. Yersinia pseudotuberculosis harbors a type IV pilus gene cluster that contributes to pathogenicity. Infect Immun 2002;70(11):6196–6205

Marketon MM, DePaolo RW, DeBord KL, Jabri B, Schneewind O. Plague bacteria target immune cells during infection. Science 2005;309(5741):1739–1741

Perry RD, Fetherston JD. Yersinia pestis-etiologic agent of plague. Clin Microbiol Rev 1997;10(1):35–66

Prentice MB, Rahalison L. Plague. Lancet 2007;369(9568):1196–1207

Pujol C, Bliska JB. Turning Yersinia pathogenesis outside in: subversion of macrophage function by intracellular yersiniae. Clin Immunol 2005;114(3):216–226

Zhou D, Han Y, Yang R. Molecular and physiological insights into plague transmission, virulence and etiology. Microbes Infect 2006;8(1):273-284 Available at: https://emergency.cdc.gov/bioterrorism/. Accessed September 2, 2019

Index